DR MEGAN ROSSI

Eat More, Live Well

Enjoy Your Favourite Food and Boost Your Gut Health with the **Diversity Diet**

Photography by Andrew Burton

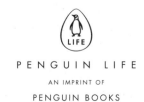

PENGUIN LIFE

AN IMPRINT OF

PENGUIN BOOKS

PENGUIN LIFE

UK | USA | Canada | Ireland | Australia
India | New Zealand | South Africa

Penguin Life is part of the Penguin Random House group of companies
whose addresses can be found at global.penguinrandomhouse.com.

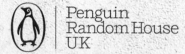

First published 2021
001

Text copyright © Dr Megan Rossi, 2021
Photography copyright © Andrew Burton, 2021
Except images on pp. 34–35, 98–99, 128–129 copyright © Shutterstock

The moral right of the author has been asserted

Printed and bound in Italy by Printer Trento
Colour origination by Altaimage, London

The authorized representative in the EEA is Penguin Random House Ireland,
Morrison Chambers, 32 Nassau Street, Dublin D02 YH68

A CIP catalogue record for this book is available from the British Library

ISBN: 978–0–241–48046–5

www.greenpenguin.co.uk

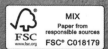

MIX
Paper from
responsible sources
FSC
www.fsc.org   FSC® C018179

Penguin Random House is committed to a
sustainable future for our business, our readers
and our planet. This book is made from Forest
Stewardship Council® certified paper.

Contents

Plant-based eating – redefined

Welcome to a delicious and sustainable way of eating that's good for you, your gut microbes and the planet. If you're looking for an easy, science-backed way to increase your energy, boost your mood, regulate your digestion, find your happy weight *and* slash your risk of chronic disease, you're in the right place. As a dietitian and research scientist, I'm here to explain why simply shifting your diet to include more plants could be the best thing you ever do for your health and happiness. And it's an approach based on facts, not fads.

This book will show you how versatile plant-based eating actually is. Forget cutting out or cutting down, I'm going to show you how – and why – *increasing* the number and range of plant foods you eat taps into the very latest scientific discoveries about how your body works best. That's right, eating *more* can improve your health, and my recipes and menu plans will show you just how easy and delicious it really is.

Whether it's something you've been thinking about for a while or a concept you've only just started hearing about, research suggests that more and more of us are interested in exploring plant-based eating. This might mean simply eating more veg meals each week; cutting down on meat, fish and other animal-derived products with meat-free Mondays; being a 'flexitarian'; or excluding some or all animal products completely, as in vegetarianism or veganism.

According to Google Trends, interest in veganism (an exclusively plant-based diet), increased sevenfold between 2014 and 2019, and it's now getting four times as many searches as vegetarian or gluten-free. The number of vegans in the UK quadrupled over this same period; and over the past six years, the number of books related to veganism has increased tenfold.

But we all know that we need to eat more veg, and there's lots of information already out there, so what's different about *this* book? Well, first of all, the science. I'm not promoting a fully vegan diet, because research doesn't necessarily support that from a health perspective (more on that in chapter 2). I'm not even suggesting you should go vegetarian, although this book is still for you if you're vegetarian or vegan. What the evidence suggests is that we could all benefit from eating *more* plants, but that doesn't necessarily have to mean *only* plants. So, rather than being about what *not* to eat, this book is all about the many varied and astounding benefits, flavour included, of basing your diet around plants. Because once they're the star attraction, trust me, you'll experience a health transformation.

My first book, *Eat Yourself Healthy,* was designed to help people identify and tackle their digestive issues and achieve great gut health. Since it was published, I've received thousands of messages from people whose health is flourishing after following the programme it sets out. I know there are lots of you out there who are on board with the idea that gut health underpins overall health. Many people also got in touch to ask for a follow up that looked more closely at exactly which foods our gut loves and why. So, this book zooms out and speaks to anyone and everyone who simply wants to eat in a way that's more aligned with what our bodies (and gut microbes) need.

And what they definitely need more of is plants.

This book is categorically not about dieting. Neither is it a trendy fad that cuts out food groups or nutrients. Instead, it's your introduction to, and inspiration for, a life-changing way of eating that brings profound, science-backed health benefits in both the short and the long term. Sure, one of those may be to do with weight management, but the benefits linked to nourishing our gut microbes go much further than that – from mood, to skin, to hormones and immunity; they are powerful little things. There is no calorie counting here, no weighing and measuring (of yourself or the foods). In fact, there's none of the cutting out you may see with other eating plans. I see this approach as enriching, not restricting; inclusive, not exclusive. More plants, more variety, more fibre, more flavour. I call it the Diversity Diet.

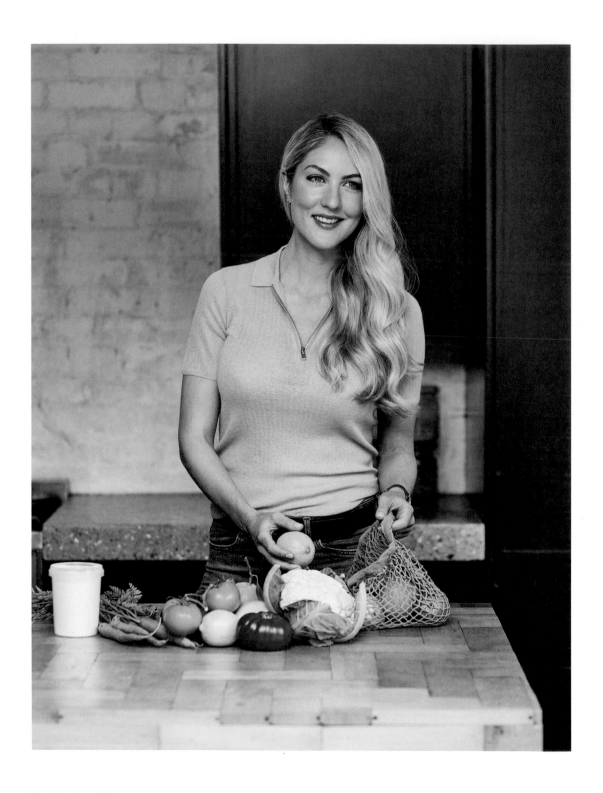

Eat More, Live Well

In *Eat Yourself Healthy*, I wrote about the vital importance of our gut microbiota. Over the past decade we have made huge leaps in our understanding of what this is and how crucial it is to our overall health. In short, the microbes (including trillions of bacteria, which we cover in more detail on page 16) that live in our gut are key to pretty much all of our body systems, and we need to make sure we have an abundant and diverse range of them to maximize our wellbeing. To do that, we need to nourish them, and what our gut microbes love most of all is an abundant and diverse range of fibre. Where does that come from? You guessed it, plants. Plant-based diversity is more than just a trend – it's based on a ground-breaking scientific discovery, and that's why it's here to stay.

I have created this book as a practical, easy route into plant-based eating, and to act as your faithful reference guide as you begin to adopt this approach in your life – however that looks for you. Over the following chapters, I'll take you through what plant-based eating is, and what constitutes a 'plant food' (prepare to be surprised at how many foods this covers) and what the Diversity Diet is all about.

Then I'll show you all the benefits of choosing this way of eating, and highlight the health impact of neglecting the power of plants. I'll give you answers to the common queries and concerns that I hear from my clients, so that you have all the information at your disposal – wherever you are on your plant-based journey. This includes my comprehensive 'toolkit' of practical evidence-based strategies, from diversity hacks to non-food exercises, all of which have successfully transformed the gut health, and overall health, of thousands of my clients.

Finally, I'll share my recipes and three different menu plans to suit a range of lifestyles. All the dishes are packed with incredible flavours and use readily available ingredients that will not just keep you fuller for longer, but boost your health and happiness from the inside out.

Now, I realize that some of you will have started your plant-based journey already. You may want to dive straight into the recipes, starting on page 133. Don't let me stop you! They're all tried-and-tested favourites that will introduce you to some delicious new foods, combinations and flavours, without a hefty price tag or the need for chef-level culinary skills. Or you might want to read up on all the background info in the next few chapters and ease yourself into the Diversity Diet more slowly, via my menu plans and gut-loving tips and tricks. Either way, I'm here to help. Whatever your reason for embarking on a plant-based way of eating, wherever you are on your journey to better health, let's do it together.

I'll be with you every step of the way.

By the end of this book, you'll know . . .

○ **What plant-based eating really means** (hint: it's not plants-only)

○ **Why fibre is the nutrient we all want more of**

○ **Why not all plant-based foods are 'healthy'**

○ **Why, when it comes to plants, diversity is key**

○ **How to get your 30 plant points a week,** and then some

○ **How to follow the Diversity Diet** and go easy on your gut

○ **How to get going today** – and keep it up for life

○ **Beyond diet** – handy lifestyle tips to nourish your gut microbes

○ **Troubleshooting** for those tricky times

○ **More than eighty tasty, plant-based recipes,** for busy people, fuelling families and sensitive guts

Ready? Let's get started . . .

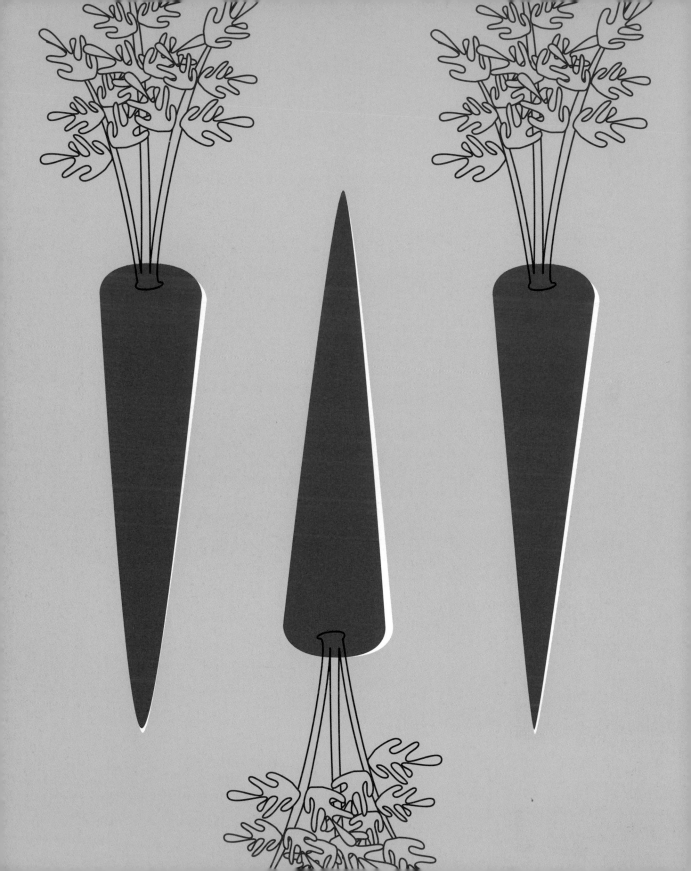

CHAPTER 1

So what *is* plant-based eating, exactly?

Is it just me, or are we all constantly bombarded with fad diets, miracle supplements and 'superfoods' that fail to live up to their claims? The 'next big thing' in health so often turns out to be just another quick fix that doesn't work long-term, and many of us have learned to be sceptical. Good health, we've been made to believe, takes hard work, sacrifice and self-restraint – and there's no such thing as a silver bullet. Except there is, kind of. Because there's one simple way to look after your gut health and reap the cascade of other benefits that it triggers: eat more plants.

How often do you hear the words 'eat' and 'more' next to each other when it comes to health advice? That's the beauty of the Diversity Diet as an evidence-based approach – *in*clusion not exclusion; adding in not cutting out.

Forget what you *think* it is . . .

Plant-based eating has become a bit of a hot topic in recent years. But where there's buzz, there's also confusion. What does plant-based eating really mean? Only eating plants? Being vegetarian? Or just eating a bit more green stuff than you did before? And is it a moral choice (*I don't eat animals*)? An environmental one (*I love Mother Earth*)? Or just the latest celeb-backed food trend (*Gwyneth told me to do it*)?

My experience with clients tells me there can be a lingering prejudice when it comes to going plant-based, whatever you believe that means. For a lot of people, it suggests a worthy attitude and bland, boring food. Some associate 'plant-based' with restriction and missing out on their favourite flavours, meals and – heaven forbid – birthday cake or grandma's famous biscuits! I'm here to reassure you that none of that applies here. This is not an extreme way of eating; quite the opposite, in fact. So let's cut the misunderstood plant world some slack, because it really does have so much to offer.

For me, the clue to defining plant-based eating is in the word 'based'. It means making plant foods the foundation of your diet. In all likelihood, it means eating more of them than you do now. But what you choose to layer on top of that – literally or ideologically – is up to you.

Just start with plants

I like to look at plant-based eating as a spectrum. I'm not one for putting labels on the way we eat, and you may well not fit within just one 'category' either, but to put plant-based eating into context, at one end you have veganism, which avoids all animal produce – meat, seafood, dairy, eggs, honey – and is focused entirely on plant foods. It's totally fine if that's what you want to do and you do it in a healthy, balanced way, which can mean a little extra work (something I touch on later, on page 87). At the other end of the plant-based eating spectrum is flexitarianism, where you eat small amounts of meat – whether that's once a day, once a week or less frequently – but still the greatest proportion of your diet comes from the plant world. Also totally fine.

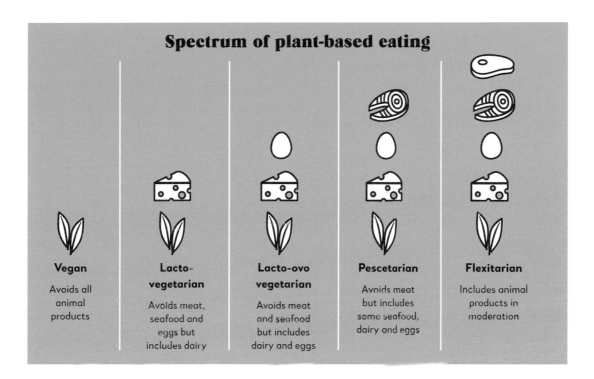

Spectrum of plant-based eating

Vegan

Avoids all animal products

Lacto-vegetarian

Avoids meat, seafood and eggs but includes dairy

Lacto-ovo vegetarian

Avoids meat and seafood but includes dairy and eggs

Pescetarian

Avoids meat but includes some seafood, dairy and eggs

Flexitarian

Includes animal products in moderation

In between, there are those who build on their plant foundation with eggs, fermented dairy, fish and so on. And you can guess what I'm going to say here . . . wherever you sit on the plant-based eating spectrum is absolutely *fine*.

In truth, including some animal foods in your diet can be a valuable way to decrease your risk of nutritional deficiencies. This is evidenced by the 'planetary health plate', developed as a result of thousands of scientific papers by a board of independent researchers from sixteen countries. The 'plate' sets out a universally healthy reference diet, which takes into account the nutritional needs and overall health of humans and, importantly, considers the environment and long-term sustainability – and guess what, the diet does include some animal foods, albeit in much smaller quantities than we eat now. So, I am in no way anti-meat. What I am, emphatically, is pro-plants.

When I say eat *more*, it's not just about quantity, but also variety. The more diversity, the better. The beauty of the Diversity Diet is it naturally makes your diet more abundant and diverse. Think 'plants' and you might immediately picture green veg and salads. But as the next chapter, along with my recipes (starting on page 133) will demonstrate, there's a wealth of flavour and colour that comes from plants – wholegrains, fruits, vegetables, nuts and seeds, legumes (beans and pulses), even herbs and spices (including tea and coffee) – out there to enjoy and fill up on.

Meet your gut microbiota . . .

Your gut microbiota, or what I call your GM, is the collective name for your gut microbes – the trillions of microorganisms, including bacteria, viruses, fungi and parasites, that live along your nine-metre digestive tract. And they can't get enough of this plant goodness. Your GM isn't just important for healthy digestion; it also, as research is showing, affects pretty much all aspects of your health, from your immunity to your skin and even your brain function (much more on this later).

Your microbes are foodies by nature. Indeed, they're actually key to *making* many of our most tongue-tinglingly flavoursome foods: chocolate, coffee, cheese, olives, soy sauce, wine. They love to sample as many different plant-based ingredients as they can. And you should let them, because the evidence shows that the more diverse your diet, the more diverse and adaptable your GM is likely to be.

Why does this matter? Intuitively, we know diversity is key to all aspects of life. It can apply to a sports team (they need defenders as much as attackers) and to our fitness (we need to work all our muscles, not just a chosen few). Or think about the resilience of rainforests – how every living organism plays its part, and upsetting that delicate ecosystem can have huge consequences.

Your gut microbes are no different. A more diverse input creates a stronger output. Think more skills and a greater support network within you. Call them your superpowers, your inner potential – however you refer to them, we're learning that they're more powerful than all our human cells combined.

Fuelled by fibre

In my first book, *Eat Yourself Healthy*, we covered that dietary fibre is essentially the backbone of plant-based foods, and it does way more than just keep you regular. We humans can't break down this type of plant-based carbohydrate during digestion, so it passes all the way into the large intestine (the final 1.5 metres of our digestive tract), where the bulk of our gut microbes live and take up that task. Another way to think of it is that fibre is one of your GM's favourite types of nutrients.

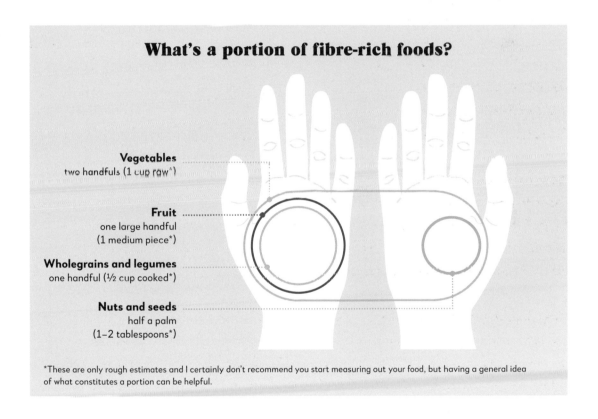

What's a portion of fibre-rich foods?

Vegetables
two handfuls (1 cup raw*)

Fruit
one large handful
(1 medium piece*)

Wholegrains and legumes
one handful (½ cup cooked*)

Nuts and seeds
half a palm
(1–2 tablespoons*)

*These are only rough estimates and I certainly don't recommend you start measuring out your food, but having a general idea of what constitutes a portion can be helpful.

Those microbes are hungry for as many types of fibre as you can feed them. And that's where this book comes in. I'll be showing you how to pack in more plant fibres than you thought possible.

Fibre facts: your at-a-glance guide to this all-important plant stuff

What is it?

A complex carbohydrate (yes, fibre is a carb!) and the all-important nutrient in plant-based foods. Unlike other carbs, such as starches and sugars, humans can't digest fibre – we simply don't make the right digestive enzymes. That's where our gut microbes come into play, they digest fibre for us.

Where is it found?

Plants! Whole plants. And there are different types of fibre found in different types of plant foods – close to a hundred, in fact – which is why diversity in your food choices is key.

What does it do?

Fibre keeps you regular by bulking out your poop and giving your gut muscles something to work with. It binds to other compounds, lowering cholesterol and preventing blood-sugar spikes. But perhaps most importantly, it feeds your GM, which breaks down fibre to produce beneficial compounds called short-chain fatty acids (SCFAs). These nourish your gut lining and have been shown to influence immunity, hormones, metabolism, your heart, brain – the list goes on (as you'll learn in chapter 4).

So why all the fuss?

Because the chances are you're missing out – and I don't want you to miss all the incredible benefits fibre brings. The recommended daily intake of fibre is 30 grams in most countries. The average intake? Well under 20 grams. Our ancestors, on the other hand, used to clock up about 100 grams a day! Now, I'm not suggesting you have to hit that, but increasing your intake by 50 per cent over time is a good place to start.

How do you get 30 grams in a day?

Around three portions of wholegrains, two pieces of fruit, five portions of veg and one to two portions of nuts, seeds or legumes per day should do it. Sounds like a lot? You'll automatically get that and more when you follow my menu plans (see page 120), without any extra thought or hassle.

Still need convincing?

Upping your fibre by just 8 grams per day is linked with a reduced risk of heart disease, type 2 diabetes, colon cancer and death from all causes. Essentially, a well-fed GM really can transform your health.

The only 'rule' is diversity

In this funny old world of social media and hashtags, many of us like to belong to a food tribe. How we choose to eat can become like an identity, a way we introduce ourselves – and something we might fear or feel guilty about deviating from. But that's not necessarily healthy. Healthy is much easier, I promise. We can ditch our quest for perfection and rigid diets, because really it doesn't seem to matter where we sit along the spectrum of plant-based eating.

What does matter is plant-based *diversity* – or how many different types of plant you can get in. Forget five a day, we're going to get you into double figures. In fact, my advice is to aim for 30 plant points every week – that's 30 different types of plant foods, which includes wholegrains, fruits, vegetables, nuts and seeds, legumes (beans and pulses) and herbs and spices (including tea and coffee).

But don't worry, I promise hitting your diversity goals is easier than you might think.

We'll take it slow, and make it fun, easy and, most importantly, flavoursome. I've convinced even the most committed meat eaters that adding more plants to their plate is a much tastier way to go – one of my most satisfying achievements to date!

Rest assured, I'm not going to leave you with just the top-level stuff. In this book we'll get down to the nitty-gritty and practical aspects – we'll look at what these foods are, how to count your plant points, how the Diversity Diet actually benefits our bodies, how we can make simple changes to our current eating habits, and also resolve any reservations you may have about going plant-based. Whether you're worried about taste, cooking skills, costs or managing a more sensitive gut, chapter 5 has you covered.

6 Principles of the Diversity Diet

1. **Mostly plants.** Make plants the base of your diet (building on this foundation with eggs, fermented dairy, fish etc. as you choose).

2. **Diversity all the way.** Aim for 30+ plant points a week, including wholegrains, fruits, vegetables, nuts and seeds, legumes, herbs and spices.

3. **Go for whole, not refined.** Opt for whole plants that have been minimally 'tampered' with or processed. More nutrients and less waste – it's a win for you, your microbes and the planet.

4. **INclusion not EXclusion.** Focus on what you're adding in, not cutting out. It's a science-backed way to transform your relationship with food.

5. **Taste, pause and enjoy.** Embrace these, and good health and digestion tend to take care of themselves. It's not just about *what* you eat, it's about *how* you eat too.

6. **Cultivate community.** See each meal as an opportunity to share, connect and learn. Because eating (and many of the associated health benefits) is about community, culture and experiences too.

And that's it! Forget the calorie counting, forget the red and green food lists, forget the inevitable restrictions that the word 'diet' typically implies. The Diversity Diet is an easy, delicious, and science-backed way of eating, governed by just six principles. Embrace these and you'll be well on your way to transforming your overall health and happiness from the inside out.

What 30 plant points actually looks like

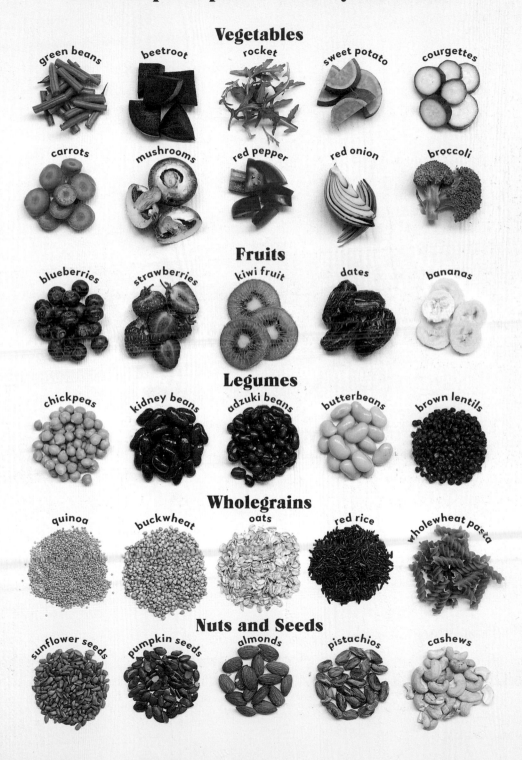

Vegetables

green beans · beetroot · rocket · sweet potato · courgettes

carrots · mushrooms · red pepper · red onion · broccoli

Fruits

blueberries · strawberries · kiwi fruit · dates · bananas

Legumes

chickpeas · kidney beans · azuki beans · butterbeans · brown lentils

Wholegrains

quinoa · buckwheat · oats · red rice · wholewheat pasta

Nuts and Seeds

sunflower seeds · pumpkin seeds · almonds · pistachios · cashews

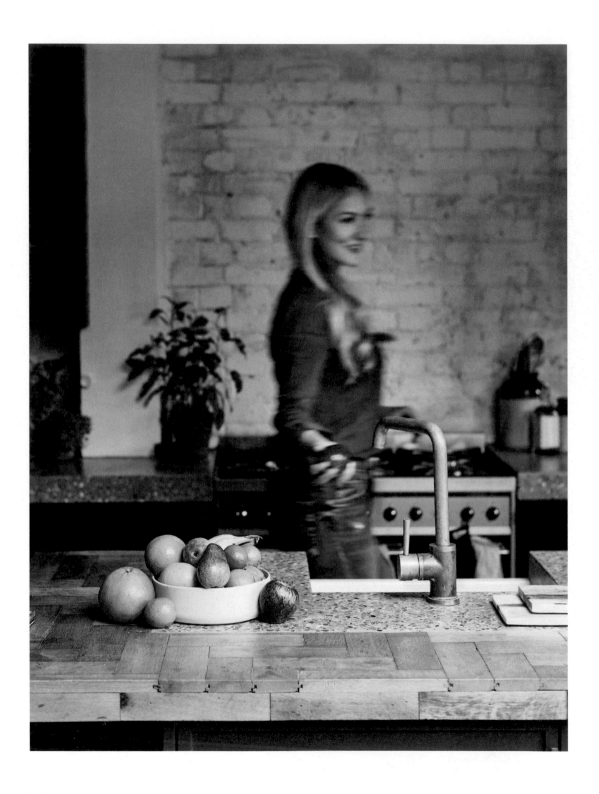

Eat More, Live Well

Learning to love plants

So the goal is a diet based mainly on plants. But what if you're just not that into them? Believe me, I've met a lot of people who weren't the biggest plant fans at first. Despite the perceived simplicity of eating (many of us can down a meal while distracted, without a thought), it's a complex affair. Still hate Brussels sprouts? Forced to eat them as a kid? Often, negative memories persist into adulthood.

But what if it's purely the taste of certain vegetables that you don't like? There are two things to consider here. First, every food can taste bad if it's not prepped right. There's a world of difference between soggy, overcooked broccoli and lightly steamed, crunchy florets roasted in soy sauce and garlic. Cooking methods matter, especially when it comes to veg – plus, I'm all about adding the right flavours to plants to make them irresistible, something we'll do plenty of in the recipes in this book

Second, the way we perceive taste is influenced by a range of factors, from the smell and texture of food to our taste buds, genes and perhaps even our microbes. Did you know, for example, that your taste buds adapt and can regenerate every ten or so days? This means a lot of your food preferences are learned, as was the case with David, whose story, on the next page, was an interesting one.

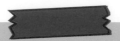

Case study

I met 29-year-old David in clinic, along with his wife, Hannah, who'd booked him in because they wanted to start trying for a baby. Hannah had read that it wasn't just the woman's diet that could impact on fertility; what the man ate mattered too. David was equally fascinated by it all.

Sat in front of me was a very drained David, who was a trainee A&E doctor coming off a run of night shifts. As we reviewed his diet, David explained that his food choices had gone downhill since he started working in A&E, and that he had fallen into the trap of getting post-shift pick-me-ups from the drive-thru of his local fast-food chain. For David, it was more about working on behaviour change, because he was all too aware of the benefits of healthy eating, having six months earlier lost his father to a diet-related heart attack at the age of sixty-two.

Together, the three of us came up with a plan that included: upping the plant-based protein source in his meal at work (we went with different legumes to increase the satiety factor); having a tasty plant-based snack in his car for his pick-me-up (see my ultimate raspberry and white choc muffins on page 161 and the prebiotic rocky road on page 281 for some you can make for yourself); and changing his route home in order to help break that habit of turning in to the drive-thru, where there was not a veg in sight.

When I saw David a few weeks on, he told me he'd 'relapsed' a few times. I reassured him it wasn't all or nothing. If he did stop off for that burger occasionally, there was no need for guilt. Instead, one simple principle applied – he was to add two different veg to the burger when he got home.

Five weeks later, a fascinating change had happened. David explained that, after weeks of forgoing the fast food for more wholesome, plant-based meals, he'd decided to treat himself with a super-sized burger one night after a particularly hard shift. It was striking how upset David looked when he recounted how, when he bit into the burger, the taste wasn't as he'd remembered. He didn't get the same kick as before.

By changing his diet, David had allowed his taste buds to change, such that the foods he used to crave no longer seemed as delicious. David remarked that the taste change was 'like magic' – except it wasn't, it was based on science, and it was something that I see happen time and time again in clinic.

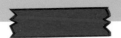

A matter of taste

So, how does this work? Well, alongside our taste-bud regeneration, we know that repeated exposure is important. Research shows you can train your taste buds by eating more of the foods you don't (think you) like, particularly for more complex flavours. Think about it – when you were younger, how many times did you take a sip of your parents' coffee or wine, or try an olive or dark chocolate, and think 'yuck'? And yet eventually you got used to the taste and now might even crave it.

Making change gradually is also key. For example, the big cereal companies have managed to remove over 40 per cent of the salt in breakfast cereals since 1998, saving the UK around 240 tonnes of salt from this one food category each year. Did their customers object? No, we didn't even notice.

My point is, our food preferences are not set in stone, and our palates can evolve if we let them.

Good for you, good for the planet . . .

Finally, let's not forget climate change. While you're feeding your inner ecosystem, you also get the satisfaction of nourishing the global one. Recent research has revealed a quarter of all global greenhouse gas emissions come from food – and more than half of those come from animal produce. What's more, cutting down your meat intake (below 100 grams per day) reduces your dietary carbon footprint (greenhouse gas emissions) by over 20 per cent. So, if you want to go green? Tip the balance in favour of plants.

In the next chapter, we'll look at how to do just that.

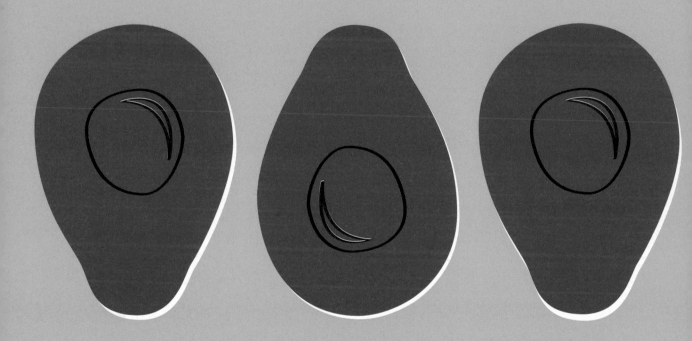

CHAPTER 2

What are plant-based foods?

Broadly speaking, plant-based foods are any foods that originate from plants. That might sound obvious – well, okay, it *is* obvious – but what I mean is it's easy just to think of the plants themselves, the leaves. Or even just to think of vegetables and fruit.

But 'plant-based' means all parts of a plant and what it produces. I'm talking roots (carrots, ginger), leaves and stems (spinach, rocket, chard), fruit (citrus, berries, apples), wholegrains (barley, oats, millet), nuts and seeds (almonds, cashews, sesame, sunflower) – both in their raw forms and everything we can make from them. When you think about plants in this way, a whole new range of produce makes itself available to you. And by proudly proclaiming plant-based foods as the foundation of your diet, you feel less like a rabbit and more like a culinary adventurer.

The Super Six

To highlight just how many plant-based foods are out there for your eating pleasure, we can divide them up into six main categories, based generally on the key nutrients they provide us and our gut microbes.

1. Wholegrains

2. Fruits

3. Vegetables

4. Nuts and seeds

5. Legumes

6. Herbs and spices

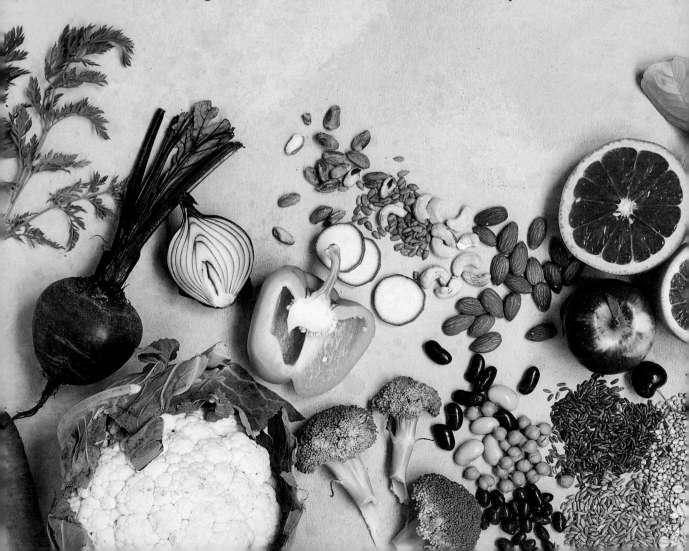

Plant points: what counts?

All your Super Six count towards your weekly plant-point goals. Here is a quick guide to adding up your plant points.

1 plant food = 1 plant point	and	1 herb or spice = ¼ plant point

- Points are given for each different variety of plant (so if you eat ten strawberries it only counts as one point).

- Different-coloured fruit and vegetables (such as green and red apples or orange, red and yellow peppers) count as a new point.

- Fresh, dried and tinned plants (always aim for no added salt and sugar) all count, so don't worry if you can only get one or the other.

- Extra virgin olive oil, tea and coffee count as ¼ point in the same way as your herbs and spices do.

- Refined plants such as fruit and vegetable juices, white grains etc. don't count, so try and stick to your whole foods as we'll cover in the following pages.

There's no need to get too caught up on portions at this stage – focus on the diversity. By having small amounts throughout the week, chances are they'll add up to a full portion overall.

How many plant points did you get today?

Here's a quick quiz for you. Think back over what you've eaten so far today (or yesterday, if it's still early in the day when you're reading this). How many plant points did you have?

Keep a note of your number, as we'll come back to this at the end of the chapter.

Not all plants are created equal

As we discussed in the last chapter, plant-based eating is a spectrum, and you don't have to eliminate all or even any animal products to consider your diet to be based on plants. Keep in mind it's not necessarily healthier to be vegan or vegetarian. When it comes to your health, the *quality* of the plant-based foods you eat is as important as the quantity.

The plant-based diet index (PDI)

To put the concept that 'plant-based' doesn't automatically equal 'healthy' to the test, a team of researchers developed the plant-based diet index (PDI). It's a way of scoring plant foods which essentially classifies them based on the level and nature of processing. The 'healthy' PDI (hPDI) positively scores high-quality whole plant foods that have been linked with health benefits. These include minimally processed wholegrains, whole fruits, vegetables, nuts and seeds, legumes, herbs and spices – aka our Super Six. In contrast, the 'unhealthy' PDI (uPDI) positively scores low-quality, highly processed plant foods that have been stripped of their whole-food goodness, such as refined grains and cereals, fruit juices, pastries and concentrated sugars such as jams and syrups.

The more **high-quality plant foods** eaten, ⬆ **hPDI score**.

The more **low-quality plant foods** eaten, ⬇ **hPDI score**.

The researchers then applied this scoring system to the diets of more than 200,000 people, who were followed for up to twenty-eight years, and what they found was pretty powerful. Those eating healthy plant foods were strongly associated with a lower risk of heart disease (those with the highest hPDI had a 25 per cent lower risk than those with the lowest hPDI). In contrast, those eating unhealthy plant foods were associated with an increased risk of heart disease (a 32 per cent increased risk in those with the highest uPDI versus the lowest uPDI).

What's more, the hPDI has been linked with gut health – which really isn't that surprising, given that whole plants are loaded with goodness for our microbes, much of which has been stripped out of the refined alternatives. When it comes to assessing a healthy plant-based diet, then, the level of processing is absolutely key. This underpins the third principle of the Diversity Diet: 'Go for whole, not refined'.

Hands up if you know someone who's vegetarian or vegan but seems to exist solely on potato crisps, margherita pizzas and highly processed meat substitutes? You may even recognize yourself. Rest assured, you're not alone. Research shows that over 50 per cent of the food (in terms of the amount of energy it provides) we eat is ultra-processed. In other words, most of the ingredients are refined parts of whole foods (such as soy protein instead of the whole soybean), combined with additives.

Someone who fitted this pattern was 24-year-old Erin:

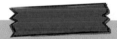

Case study

I met Erin in clinic, six months after she had decided to go vegan. From both a health and an animal-cruelty perspective, she believed this was the right thing for her. But Erin recounted to me that, four months in, things didn't feel quite right. Not only had she gained 5 kilograms, but she was experiencing brain fog and her skin had started to break out more frequently (and not just around her periods like before). She'd also caught two colds that had sent her to bed, despite previously being rather proud of her resilient immune system.

As I reviewed Erin's diet before and after turning vegan, it was clear what had happened. She had fallen into the trap of relying on those convenient animal-food lookalikes – we're talking vegan cheese slices, imitation chicken nuggets, no-beef burgers, plant-protein shakes. Not only was she having fewer whole plant foods than she'd had previously, she was overeating ultra-processed vegan alternatives in an attempt to compensate for the flavour of animal foods she missed.

So what did we do? We switched out a lot of the processed foods for less-processed alternatives. These swaps became really easy once she learned what they were: cashew cheese instead of vegan cheese (see the loaded vegan nachos on page 231); whole-plant burgers instead of additive-laden soy protein patties (check out the smoky beet burger on page 213), and whole plant-based sources of protein such as tofu and nuts instead of refined protein powders ➝

(try the Snickers smoothie bowl on page 293). We prioritized nourishing her inner community of gut microbes, while also celebrating the array of flavours plants have to offer. As for the animal produce, I left that up to Erin.

When I reviewed her progress eight weeks later, she explained that she had decided to reintroduce some animal foods, but kept it to just fermented dairy that was sourced from a local farm, as well as small amounts of local and organic meats. Erin also shared her verdict on my beet burgers: 'Cheaper, deceivingly quick to make and they bring a whole other category of flavour to my plate – I'm sold!'

And the health outcome? Erin's weight and skin returned to her pre-vegan days and she reported: 'I feel better – inside and out – than ever before.' All from just a few simple tweaks.

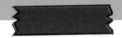

What do healthy plant-based foods provide?

Let's take a look at the beneficial nutrients each plant group offers. The table on page 33 includes the three macronutrients (carbohydrates, proteins, fats) as well as key essential micronutrients (vitamins and minerals). I've included the main nutrients each group can be considered a good source of, as well as other notable nutrients that contribute to your dietary intake.

It's no secret that you could go into any pharmacy, supermarket or health food store and buy each micronutrient listed in the table to take in supplement form – whether as a single vitamin or mineral or as part of a multi-nutrient formula. And there is an argument for supporting your diet with certain supplements at certain times in your life, such as if you're pregnant or you're not including all food groups in the case of a vegan diet (see page 87). But here's why popping pills is no substitute for a plant-based diet . . .

There's a wealth of vitamins and minerals contained in each plant food, and these really are team players. They act in synergy with each other – one helping another to be absorbed – and with all the different types of fibre that plant foods contain (remember, fibre is our GM's must-have). This explains why the majority of studies show that micronutrients entering the body through food are generally more beneficial than those in supplement form. The sum of a plant's nutrients is way greater than its parts.

Key nutrients found in the different plant-based food groups

	Wholegrains	Fruit	Vegetables	Nuts and seeds	Legumes
Main distinguishing nutrients	✓ Carbohydrate ✓ Fibre ✓ Manganese ✓ Selenium	✓ Fibre ✓ Vitamin C	✓ Fibre ✓ Folate (B9) ✓ Vitamin A* ✓ Vitamin C ✓ Vitamin K	✓ Fat ✓ Long-chain omega-3 fatty acids ✓ Magnesium ✓ Manganese ✓ Vitamin E	✓ Fibre ✓ Protein ✓ Folate (B9) ✓ Iron ✓ Phosphorus ✓ Thiamine (B1)
Other significant nutrients	✓ Protein ✓ Iron ✓ Magnesium ✓ Niacin (B3) ✓ Phosphorus ✓ Thiamine (B1) ✓ Zinc	✓ Carbohydrate ✓ Folate (B9) ✓ Manganese ✓ Potassium ✓ Vitamin A*	✓ Carbohydrate ✓ Iron ✓ Magnesium ✓ Manganese ✓ Niacin (B3) ✓ Pantothenic acid (B5) ✓ Potassium ✓ Pyridoxine (B6) ✓ Riboflavin (B2)	✓ Fibre ✓ Protein ✓ Iron ✓ Niacin (B3) ✓ Phosphorus ✓ Pyridoxine (B6) ✓ Selenium ✓ Thiamine (B1) ✓ Zinc	✓ Carbohydrate ✓ Magnesium ✓ Manganese ✓ Phosphorus ✓ Pyridoxine (B6) ✓ Selenium ✓ Zinc

*In the form of beta-carotene, which the body converts to vitamin A.

This is just a general guide. Foods within each group vary, and that is the beauty of plant-based diversity.

What about herbs and spices? They don't typically provide us with significant amounts of macro- or micronutrients. But that's no reason to disregard them – they still have plenty to offer! Read on and you'll discover the wonders of phytochemicals . . .

Phytochemicals – a whole new world of plant power

The benefits of plant-based foods go well beyond macro- and micronutrients; they are full of phytochemicals too. Phytochemicals are essentially plant chemicals, many of which have been shown to have a host of beneficial effects in the body. There are literally tens of thousands of different phytochemicals, each with different functions. It's these phytochemicals that give plants much of their colour, flavour, aroma and texture. While there's still a lot we don't yet know about phytochemicals, here are five ways that they have been shown to benefit us, with examples of plant sources in bold (based on test-tube studies):

1. Antioxidant and inflammation-quenching powers

These protect our cells against damaging compounds known as free radicals, which can play a role in the ageing process and also cancer formation, among many other conditions. Phytochemicals with antioxidant activity include allyl sulfides (**onions, leeks, garlic**), carotenoids (**carrots, tomatoes, peppers**) and flavonoids (**teas, berries, kale**).

2. Hormone regulators

Some are hormones themselves, such as melatonin (**black rice, pistachios, peppers**); others act similarly to hormones, like phytoestrogens (**soy, broccoli, oranges**); and many interact with hormones, such as indoles and glucosinolates (**cabbages, cauliflower, Brussels sprouts**), which have been shown to reduce the production of cancer-related hormones.

3. Barrier warriors

This protective trait prevents invaders from attaching to our cell walls, including our urinary tract. Take the proanthocyanidins found in **cranberries**; these barrier warriors are to thank for helping to prevent the attachment of pathogens that cause urinary tract infections.

4. Immune supporters

Several phytochemicals have been shown to directly interact with the army of immune chemicals in our body. The flavonoid family (**peaches, grapes, kidney beans**), of which there are over 6,000 types, are well-known immune supporters.

5. Brain messengers

Many are also linked with the nervous system, including dietary neurotransmitters (communication chemicals) such as gamma aminobutyric acid or GABA (**peas, tomatoes, buckwheat**), serotonin (**pomegranates, potatoes, hazelnuts**) and dopamine (**bananas, avocados, aubergines**).

While phytochemicals are technically not essential for human survival (unlike micronutrients), they're thought to explain much of the difference between those of us who are just 'surviving' versus those who really are 'thriving'. A diet packed with a wide range of phytochemicals is far more likely to mean a happy, healthy and energized person.

And you thought it was just an apple . . .

They say an apple a day keeps the doctor away and, sure enough, there's a whole pharmacy of amazing ingredients hiding in and under that peel. Let's take a look at how much bang you get for every bite. (And remember, this is just a humble apple – I could provide thousands of examples of plant foods with similarly impressive, yet strikingly different, credentials.)

Yes, apples are a source of carbohydrates, including fibre, and vitamins and minerals, but break it down further and there are around 300 different phytochemicals packed into that little sphere.

As well as feeding your gut bacteria with all the fibres and various phytochemicals, each apple has also been shown to contain some 100 million bacteria of its own too. So eating an apple may very well help make your GM abundant and diverse in more ways than one.

Just as there are lots of varieties of apple – more than 7,500 in fact – there will be variations in the nutrient profile. These days, however, most supermarket-bought apples are based on just a handful of varieties, bred for their sweetness, most of which contain a lower phytochemical punch compared to that of the older varieties. Additionally, wonky imperfect fruit and veg have been shown to contain more phytochemicals. That's because they have faced more stress and, in response, they produce more of these great chemicals. What doesn't kill you makes you stronger, right? It's the same for plants! So embrace diversity in your apple choices – show some love to the weird and wonky ones!

An apple is just one example of a plant-based food and all the nutrient diversity to be found within. Now expand this to all the other plant-based foods you eat, filled with countless different phytochemicals, and suddenly your diet looks like some sort of magical plant pharmacy!

This is why I'm not a big fan of the term 'superfood' – to me all plants are pretty fantastic.

The apple pharmacy

Here's just a taster of what you might find

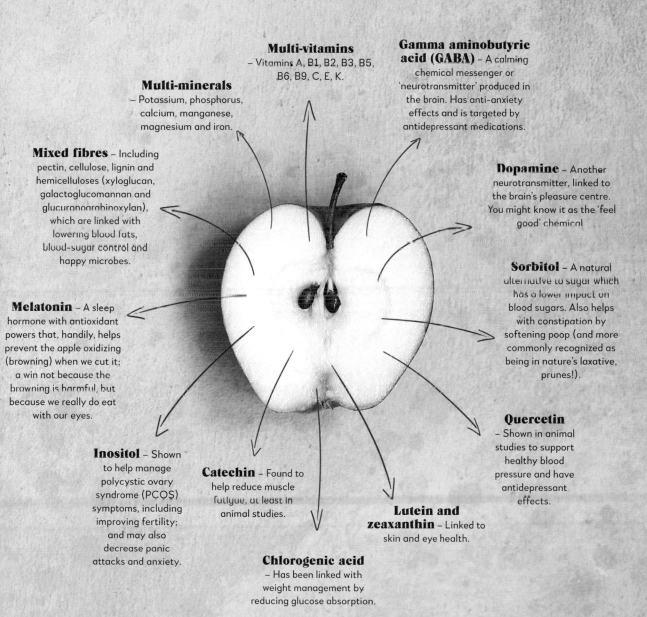

Multi-vitamins – Vitamins A, B1, B2, B3, B5, B6, B9, C, E, K.

Gamma aminobutyric acid (GABA) – A calming chemical messenger or 'neurotransmitter' produced in the brain. Has anti-anxiety effects and is targeted by antidepressant medications.

Multi-minerals – Potassium, phosphorus, calcium, manganese, magnesium and iron.

Mixed fibres – Including pectin, cellulose, lignin and hemicelluloses (xyloglucan, galactoglucomannan and glucuronoarabinoxylan), which are linked with lowering blood fats, blood-sugar control and happy microbes.

Dopamine – Another neurotransmitter, linked to the brain's pleasure centre. You might know it as the 'feel good' chemical

Sorbitol – A natural alternative to sugar which has a lower impact on blood sugars. Also helps with constipation by softening poop (and more commonly recognized as being in nature's laxative, prunes!).

Melatonin – A sleep hormone with antioxidant powers that, handily, helps prevent the apple oxidizing (browning) when we cut it; a win not because the browning is harmful, but because we really do eat with our eyes.

Quercetin – Shown in animal studies to support healthy blood pressure and have antidepressant effects.

Inositol – Shown to help manage polycystic ovary syndrome (PCOS) symptoms, including improving fertility; and may also decrease panic attacks and anxiety.

Catechin – Found to help reduce muscle fatigue, at least in animal studies.

Lutein and zeaxanthin – Linked to skin and eye health.

Chlorogenic acid – Has been linked with weight management by reducing glucose absorption.

Surviving vs thriving

Recent years have seen a worrying trend for 'no need to eat' meal replacements. You know, those drinks marketed at high-flying execs who want all their nutrition without having to stop for meals. Typically, the drinks include all your essential micronutrients, the three macronutrients plus one of the near-hundred types of fibres, as well as an array of additives such as emulsifiers and sweeteners. To me, they epitomize surviving without thriving – something I noted in 32-year-old Harry:

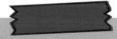

Case study

Harry was an IT executive. He was the definition of 'work hard and play hard', but as the years rolled by and the work pressure stacked up, he explained, everything was feeling more difficult. Preparing meals, going to the gym, dating, late nights, early mornings – something had to give. One of his colleagues mentioned these meal-replacement drinks so he thought he'd give them a go. One less thing to worry about.

Three months later, Harry was sat in front of me. He couldn't quite understand why, although all his blood work had come back normal (he was surviving), he felt even worse now despite all that time saved by not cooking, shopping and chewing. I explained to him it was likely to be those missing phytochemicals and fibres. He jumped at the idea of a solution: 'Where can I buy them?' And that's when I had to break it to him . . .

The thing about phytochemicals and dietary fibres is that Mother Nature has them hanging over us; we haven't yet figured out how to actually manufacture most of them. To start thriving, Harry was going to have to realize that plant-based foods work in synergy – and he needed to make some time for real food.

And, sure enough, after returning to whole food and upping the diversity of plants, using the hacks on page 96, as well as managing his stress with the strategies on page 116, he was soon back to his energized self.

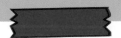

Why plants = protein

Protein is one of the three macronutrients and is essential for growing and repairing our body's tissues and making enzymes, hormones and other chemicals, as well as providing some energy. Yet often when we think about protein, we just think of meat.

That's probably because animal products – not just meat, but fish, eggs and dairy – are what are called 'complete' proteins. This means they contain all nine essential building blocks of protein (aka amino acids) that our bodies can't make on their own. So you could call animal produce an easy win, protein-wise. But getting protein from plants really isn't much harder – you just need a range of sources to ensure you get those essential nine.

Newsflash: several studies show vegans and vegetarians actually get plenty of protein (recommended to be around 1 gram per kilogram of body weight daily). Ignore the outdated stereotype of 'hippie' vegans as sandal-wearing weaklings; I've known many a plant-based bodybuilder or endurance athlete – I imagine you probably do too.

Sure, if you want to build muscle on a vegan diet, you might have to be a bit clever about the plant sources of protein you consume. But for the vast majority of us non-athletes, just making sure we eat a variety of plant-based foods is all it takes. Yes, a plate of lettuce leaves and cherry tomatoes only contains a couple of grams of protein, but switch that up for a diverse salad such as my *reinvented* couscous salad (page 208) and you'll be getting around 30 grams of plant-protein per portion, not to mention added flavour.

Ask Google and you'll probably read that rice and beans are the best combo to get the right mix of those essential amino acids. But because you know by now that we're all about diversity, I can assure you that any mix of wholegrains and legumes together will help fill the amino acid gaps to deliver a 'complete' protein – and of course, any other plant-based foods you want to throw in. The more the merrier; variety is key.

Stick to this principle and you won't need to bore yourself trying to find the perfect combination; it will just come naturally.

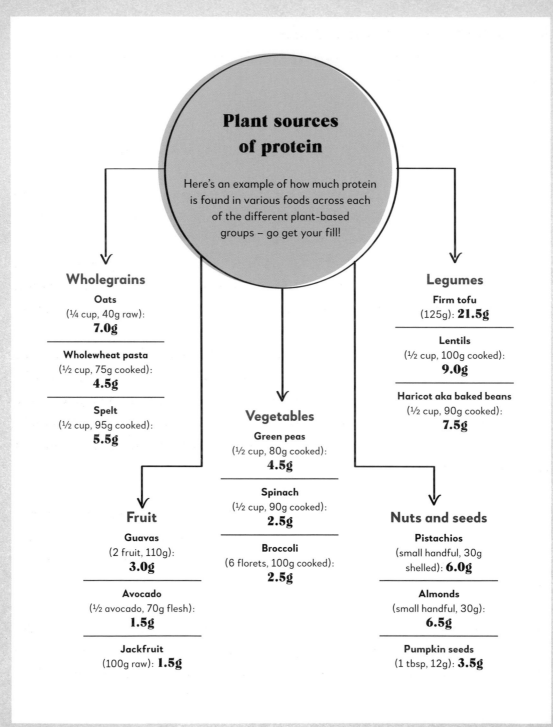

Plant sources of protein

Here's an example of how much protein is found in various foods across each of the different plant-based groups – go get your fill!

Wholegrains

Oats
(¼ cup, 40g raw):
7.0g

Wholewheat pasta
(½ cup, 75g cooked):
4.5g

Spelt
(½ cup, 95g cooked):
5.5g

Fruit

Guavas
(2 fruit, 110g):
3.0g

Avocado
(½ avocado, 70g flesh):
1.5g

Jackfruit
(100g raw): **1.5g**

Vegetables

Green peas
(½ cup, 80g cooked):
4.5g

Spinach
(½ cup, 90g cooked):
2.5g

Broccoli
(6 florets, 100g cooked):
2.5g

Legumes

Firm tofu
(125g): **21.5g**

Lentils
(½ cup, 100g cooked):
9.0g

Haricot aka baked beans
(½ cup, 90g cooked):
7.5g

Nuts and seeds

Pistachios
(small handful, 30g
shelled): **6.0g**

Almonds
(small handful, 30g):
6.5g

Pumpkin seeds
(1 tbsp, 12g): **3.5g**

Data source: US Department of Agriculture

Remember those plant points?

At the beginning of this chapter I asked you to add up your plant points from across the day. So, how did you score?

I mentioned in chapter 1 that I recommend people aim for 30 – yes, 30 – different plants over the course of a week. So keep counting for seven days and see what your baseline is.

Why this target? The '5-a-day' rule can be a good place to start – but it totally ignores the trillions of microbes living in our gut. They all need different types of plants to flourish.

Where does the '30 a week' come from? It's fuelled by research that I've then tested out in clinic. One of the key studies demonstrated that people who ate at least 30 different plant-based foods a week had more diverse gut microbes than people who ate less than 10.

I think it's easy to kid ourselves into thinking we eat a wide variety of foods when really we tend to stick to the same old favourites. Modern life doesn't help – many of us just reorder the same supermarket delivery, week in, week out. When was the last time you strolled round a farmers' market, or even just looked at what the corner-shop grocer had in stock? I get that we're creatures of habit and convenience, and I'll admit that I am the same. But our GM needs us to shake it up a bit.

Make your 'journey to 30' fun. Stick the plant points planner from page 130 on your fridge and record each new plant point. Go out of your way to find new plant varieties to sample. Kids love challenges like this, and why not get friends, family or work colleagues involved too?

See every meal as an opportunity to add something extra, try something new. There are literally thousands of plants and flavours just waiting for you and your gut microbes to discover them. (Oh, and I say 30 – but once you start on your Diversity Diet journey, don't let me stop you there!)

Gut 101: a mini masterclass on your all-important GM

If you've read my first book, *Eat Yourself Healthy*, chances are you'll already be clued up and have bonded with your 'inner universe' of microbes. But if not, here's a little recap of why these beneficiaries of our plant-based eating are so deserving . . .

First up, we are more microbe than human. Yes, you read that correctly – there are more of them living in us than human cells. There are trillions of microbes that live on and in our bodies – in mini ecosystems in our mouths, our reproductive organs, our lungs, on our skin – although the vast majority are housed in the large intestine, and this is known as our gut microbiota (GM).

You may have grown up thinking of microbes such as bacteria, fungi, viruses and parasites as enemies to be eliminated, but in truth we need them to survive. Terms like 'friendly bacteria' are equally confusing, because really, apart from a small subset of inherently harmful microbes (including SARS-CoV-2, the virus behind COVID-19), there's no such thing as 'good' or 'bad' microbes. It's all about how they're balanced.

When it comes to your GM, the technical term for an imbalance of microbes is 'dysbiosis'. But the trouble is, because everyone's GM is unique, it's not possible right now to say exactly what the ultimate balance looks like. What we do know, however, is that when things are out of whack, poor health can result.

Gut glossary

Microbes

The smallest living organisms we know of; too small in fact to see with the naked eye, we need a microscope. This explains their scientific name, *micro*organisms. The most common include bacteria, viruses and fungi. They come in all shapes and sizes, although bacteria are far larger than viruses, around 10 to 100 times.

Microbiota

The community of microbes (you can think of them as the 'members' of our inner gut club). One of the most densely populated microbial communities on earth, far exceeding that of soil and the ocean. Together, they weigh around 200 grams.

Metabolome

The handy by-products, such as vitamins and other chemicals, that our microbes produce as they go about their job, including digesting all that fibre. (Using the club analogy, think the members' voices and belongings.)

Microbiome

The whole environment, including the microbes and the things they produce (not just the members and their things, but the whole club).

What does our GM do for us?

We know that, generally speaking, the greater the diversity of our GM, the better our overall health and resistance to infection. I always come back to that sports team analogy – you need a breadth of skills to be at the top of your game. And with so many different types of microbe out there (scientists estimate there are tens of thousands of strains of unique bacteria that can dwell in the gut), it's no surprise that we each have a distinct combination within us. Our GM is unique to us, like our fingerprints. Identical twins may share the same human genes, environment and lifestyle, but their GM will always be different.

So long as it's well supported (that's where this book comes in), our inner universe is a hive of activity, working super-hard at tasks like:

✓ **Munching up fibre** and phytochemicals from the plants we eat.
✓ **Making vitamins** (K and the different Bs), amino acids, hormones and chemical messengers.
✓ **Training our immune system.**
✓ **Activating and deactivating medicines** and toxins (this explains why, at least in part, people can respond in different ways to the same medications).
✓ **Making chemicals that strengthen** the gut barrier, helping to balance blood sugars, lower blood fats and regulate appetite.
✓ **Communicating with our brain,** skin, liver, thyroid, heart and just about every organ in the human body.
✓ **Protecting us against** a proliferation of harmful microbes.
✓ **Assisting gut movement** and function.

In other words, a thriving GM can optimize digestion, immunity, metabolism, hormones, brain function and gene expression (turning our genes 'on and off', affecting what scientists previously thought was our 'destiny'). I don't know about you, but with them having this responsibility, I think we owe it to these microbes to give them as much support as we can.

Whether you think of your GM as your inner universe, Tamagotchi, pet, friend or simply untapped potential, the next time you sit down to a meal, it's worth acknowledging you're never just eating for one.

The empowering news is that so much of our GM's health and happiness is in our control. There are many ways we can look after our GM, in terms of what we eat and how we treat it (with things like sleep, stress and even exercise, which we'll touch on in chapter 6). In fact, our diet and lifestyle choices actually have a much bigger effect on how healthy our GM is than our genetics do. And so far, research indicates that people who consume high-fibre diets made up of a wide range of whole plant-based foods from the Super Six typically have the greatest GM diversity and stability. This was the main driving force behind me writing this book – to spread this landmark discovery beyond the research bubble and help as many people as possible to embrace the far-reaching benefits of the Diversity Diet. And I hope, after reading this book and experiencing it for yourself, you'll feel equally compelled to share it too.

CHAPTER 3

Why is going plant-based so important?

My life's work has been devoted to looking at the impact of nutrition on human health, and, let me tell you, what we eat has a *huge* impact – huge! Food is life. So the types of food we eat affect our quality of life. But if you look at our collective health, something's got to give.

All the research I immerse myself in, all the convincing evidence, points to the power of plant-based foods to help us lead healthier lives. This is life-altering stuff, and something we can so easily do to safeguard ourselves against a whole host of lifestyle diseases. Given the relatively simple adjustments involved in making your diet plant-based (remember, it doesn't have to mean cutting out all animal products, and no foods are completely off limits), it's got to be worth taking this seriously. Most of us are not taking the best care of our health – and yet with a few easy changes we can, such as by switching half the meat in your pasta sauce for a tin of legumes (see page 96 for more switches) or your standard rocky road for my prebiotic version (page 281).

The hard-hitting facts

We're facing a mental-health crisis – especially in the modern world, where stress and anxiety are rife. This matters because mental health is one of the main causes of overall disease worldwide; for example, depression is one of the primary drivers of disability. With one in six of us suffering a mental health issue over the past week alone, these aren't statistics to be ignored, and thankfully they're something we can change.

The same goes for many other chronic diseases. UK diagnoses of diabetes have doubled over the past twenty years. Rates of type 2 diabetes in particular are soaring, along with those for autoimmune diseases and conditions linked to inflammation. These include allergies, rheumatoid arthritis, ulcerative colitis and Crohn's, chronic fatigue, fibromyalgia, overactive or underactive thyroid, and many, many more. And that's without touching on heart disease and many cancers. In fact, from 1993 to 2018 the percentage of people at 'very high' risk of developing a chronic disease due to their diet and lifestyle doubled, from 14 per cent to 28 per cent of women and 11 per cent to 22 per cent of men.

Humans are living longer – United Nations records show that in 1960 the average global life expectancy was 52.5 and today it's 72. But according to a 2018 study published in the journal *Age and Ageing*, these life expectancy gains will be spent mostly burdened with four or more diseases. Where's the fun in extra years if we're not happy or healthy?

As many as six in ten of us are living with a chronic disease (like heart disease, mental health conditions, metabolism issues), and four in ten have two or more. Most shockingly, in 2017 there were approximately 11 million deaths and 255 million disability-adjusted life years (meaning people are alive but disabled with disease) attributed to poor diet.

These statistics are hard to hear, but the good news is that less than 20 per cent of chronic diseases seem to be down to our genetics alone, which means that the other 80 per cent are determined by our environment and can be influenced by how we live. In fact, all the conditions we've talked about can be affected, at least in part, by diet. And they have all been linked to GM dysbiosis, something all too common in our modern societies.

In fact, our GM is linked to most, if not all, of the lifestyle diseases we face today. The more diverse our GM, the greater protection we seem to have from more than seventy chronic conditions. Evidence shows that our GM typically alters with age, exposing us to dysbiosis and the ensuing inflammation that's the root of many of these conditions. But it's not a life sentence. Remember, we can dictate much of our GM diversity by how we treat it, and therefore we have the power to stave off much of this 'inflammageing'.

The human microbiome is considered the biggest emerging area of research in medical and nutritional science of the past century. A major discovery is happening right before our eyes and revolutionizing our health. Although yes we don't know the exact nature of all the links with various diseases, and there is still more research to be done, what I can say for sure is that improving our gut health has been shown to improve our general health and happiness in enough studies to have the scientific world convinced that targeting our GM is a game-changer for our health. And, according to the scientific evidence, fibre-filled plant-based diversity is the way to fuel just that.

What are we eating?

With all the advancements in technology over the last fifty years, it has become cheaper and easier to eat processed foods instead of feeding our gut microbes with the vast array of plants they – and we – need in order to thrive. While an estimated 300,000 edible plant species are available to humans, more than half of our global energy needs are met by just four: rice, potatoes, wheat and maize. Many of us have become accustomed to thinking that sticking to these four types each day is 'normal', yet the science, the surging rates of chronic diseases and the way our ancestors ate are certainly telling us a different story.

What we need is to grow a more diverse range of microbes within us – a sure sign of optimal gut health and a reduced risk of so many of these lifestyle diseases. And how we do that is by reaching beyond just those four plants, to the thousands of other plant-based foods on offer.

4 reasons to get diversifying:

1. **A lower risk of nutritional deficiencies** – in the last chapter I talked about all those micronutrients and phytochemicals in plants. The more variety you eat, the lower your chance of becoming deficient. Each food provides different essential nutrients. Skip it and you miss out.

2. **Greater pleasure in food** – a more varied diet not only introduces a whole host of nutrients to your plate, it brings amazing tastes to your palate, too. We'll get creative with the Diversity Diet in chapter 6, so you'll soon be enjoying a richness of aromas, flavours and textures. Why does this matter? Because enjoying our food has linked to longevity, plus studies demonstrate it also has a positive impact on digestion.

3. **Better overall nutrition** – thanks to the fact many nutrients found in plant foods work together to have an additive benefit. There are so many great examples of where consuming one nutrient helps your absorption of another, see examples on page 51. A limited diet misses out on so much of this teamwork.

4. **A more diverse GM** – it's not just better nutrition for you, but your gut microbes too. The research shows that the more diverse the nutrients you supply your microbes (from the plants you eat – think fibres, prebiotics, phytochemicals) the more diverse your GM becomes. That is, the greater the support network within you.

Food pairings that enhance nutrition

Eating for sun protection

Fat increases the absorption of lycopene – a plant chemical with antioxidant powers that can help protect us against sun damage (no skipping that SPF though). You could eat one lycopene-rich tomato; or you could slice it up and have it with some gut-loving extra virgin olive oil or avocado – easily and naturally upping the amount of lycopene available for your skin to take on board.

Do you need more iron?

It can be harder to get enough iron if you don't eat meat. Unless you happen to know that vitamin C increases the amount of non-haem iron (found in plant foods) you absorb. It's as easy as adding some vitamin C-rich peppers to that lentil dish, dipping pepper crudités in hummus, or squeezing lemon juice over a salad of dark green leafy veg (see the courgette and hazelnut salad on page 184).

Like turmeric in a curry?

Who doesn't. But be sure to add a few turns of the pepper mill too. Curcumin, the active ingredient in turmeric, has been shown to have an anti-inflammatory effect in humans – although we'd need it in high doses. So it's helpful that in the presence of piperine, contained in black pepper, our body's ability to absorb curcumin increases by 2,000 per cent! (My spicy red lentil bowl is on page 240.)

One for strong bones.

Sun-drenched mushrooms (yes, they're a thing – and high in vitamin D as a result) go nicely with some calcium-set tofu. Or have some salmon (oily fish, another good source of vitamin D) with spring greens (try the orange-glazed roasted salmon on page 226). Each will boost your vitamin D intake. And being D-sufficient has been shown to increase your absorption of calcium by around 50 per cent. They're both key for a healthy skeleton.

Maxing out on magnesium

Prebiotic foods – rich in the types of fibre that feed your GM, such as inulin – are known to boost your magnesium absorption. Take advantage by combining seeds and dates (try the stuffed dates – four ways, on page 165), or nuts with artichoke (like in the creamy dairy-free linguine on page 225).

Building muscle with plants

Get your complete set of protein building blocks (aka amino acids) by combining wholegrains with legumes, or legumes with nuts or seeds. Try freekeh and mixed beans (see the Mediterranean hug soup on page 221), or black beans with cashew cheese (check out the loaded vegan nachos on page 231).

Restrictive diets = sensitive stomachs

Food sensitivities are at an all-time high. If you don't think you have some sort of food intolerance yourself, I'll bet you know plenty of people who do. Whether the perceived trigger is gluten, wheat, garlic, onion, yeast, or any other food or group, it can become problematic because it results in restrictive diets. Here's the thing – often food intolerances or sensitivities are exacerbated by and even triggered by dietary restrictions.

You know the saying 'you are what you eat'? That's never more true than with your GM. Your microbes adapt according to what foods you eat. For example, if your diet is high in meat and processed foods and low in whole plant foods, say hello to a tipping of the bacteria balance to a GM profile that is not only linked with diseases such as bowel cancer, but also the reduced ability to digest plants. That's because it's not our human cells that digest fibre, it's our microbes, as we touched on in chapter 1. When diverse, our GM is able to produce hundreds of enzymes that break down the many different types of fibres and plant chemicals found in our plant foods. But if your diet is restricted, this means that only a minority group of microbes will thrive, and in turn dominate the community, while other skilful bacteria will be left to starve and eventually die out, narrowing the range of microbes you have.

Diversity breeds diversity. So all these restrictive diets often touted as the key to health and weight loss – paleo, low carb, *no* carb – can be detrimental in the long term. If we starve our GM, when we then eat a bowl of plants, we lack many of the microbes (and therefore their enzymes) needed to digest the different fibres efficiently. This inefficient digestion can in turn trigger gut symptoms such as bloating, excess gas and altered poops.

Now, I'm not saying go out and gorge on the very foods that trigger gut symptoms for you – far from it. What I am saying is keep in mind that no plant food (unless you have a properly diagnosed allergy or coeliac disease) should be off the menu long-term.

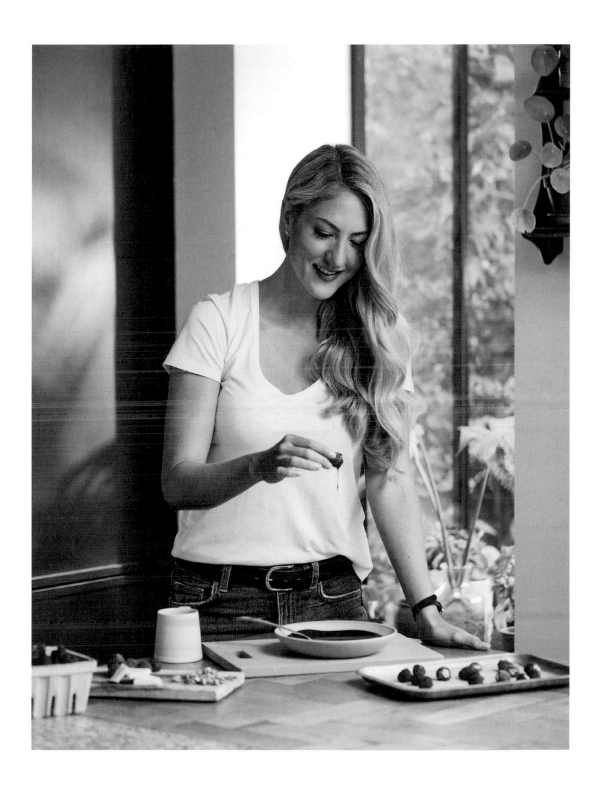

The magic of our gut microbes is that you can generally increase tolerance to plant foods you feel sensitive to. The key is to introduce them gradually and slowly, broadening your exposure and teaching your gut microbes to digest them. And, in turn, this will help to repopulate your GM and increase its diversity. It's like how we build our immunity through coming into contact with germs in smaller doses to build our tolerance, rather than living in a bubble.

If you are advised by a dietitian to follow an exclusion diet to find the food you feel intolerant to, the goal should typically involve this gradual reintroduction, not permanent elimination. This is something people – doctors included – often get wrong when it comes to irritable bowel syndrome (IBS) and the low-FODMAP diet, and people can end up getting stuck following the restriction stage of the diet for years. (Not familiar with the low-FODMAP diet? Check out page 128.) Instead, the low-FODMAP diet should include a three-stage approach: restriction, reintroduction and personalization.

The restriction stage eliminates certain foods – including garlic, onions, apples and most legumes – that are ordinarily loved by your GM. This stage of the diet should only be followed for a maximum of eight weeks, so that you don't starve off and unbalance your GM long-term. In fact, mine several other research groups have shown that extended restriction leads to a reduction in beneficial microbes such as Bifidobacteria, and it's these bacteria that have been linked to a decrease in some IBS symptoms. Go figure!

After the restriction stage, the high-FODMAP foods are gradually reintroduced. Simply put, after a little gut rest, by refeeding and fertilizing your body in small amounts, the gut gets better at tolerating former triggers.

Gut health issues and sensitivities are something that more and more of us are experiencing every year. But please don't suffer in silence. Get the help you deserve. For more information and evidence-based strategies, take a look at my website or read my first book, *Eat Yourself Healthy*. And if you know that you are sensitive to certain foods – don't worry, plant-based eating is possible for you too. I have designed the Sensitive Guts menu plan on page 126 to help ease your way into eating more plants at a pace that works for you. All of these recipes can be made FODMAP-lite with a few switches or by watching the portion size. I've marked them as FODMAP-lite in the book, with this icon at the top of the page: ⊜ And I have explained the necessary tweaks at the end of the book on pages 304–308, so be sure to check that out if this applies to you.

Plants as medicine

Did you know around a quarter of drugs prescribed worldwide are plant-derived? Just another reason not to underestimate the power of plants. They include aspirin (from willow bark), opiates such as morphine and codeine (from poppies), the heart medication digoxin (from foxgloves) and the antimalarial quinine (from the bark of a cinchona tree).

Now, I wouldn't go as far as saying food is medicine – that would be doing both a disservice, as they're very different. Modern medicine can be life-saving and I certainly wouldn't advise people to just replace their prescribed medication with eating these plants. That said, plant power is real, and nourishing our bodies with plenty of plant goodness can have a profound impact on our health, helping to manage conditions and prevent disease.

A final thought

Sure, our health has seen better days. But the good news is we know more now about *why* and *what* we can do about it than at any other time in human history.

Modern diets are simply not good enough. The range of foods we eat is too narrow; our choices are too processed – and this combination is limiting our health potential. But there is a solution: Whole. Diverse. Plants.

We have science on our side, so let's exploit what we know about our GM and do our best to optimize it.

Tip
Some of our microbiome is passed on just as our genes are. By eating more plants now, you won't just be positively affecting your own health – you'll be paying it forward to future generations.

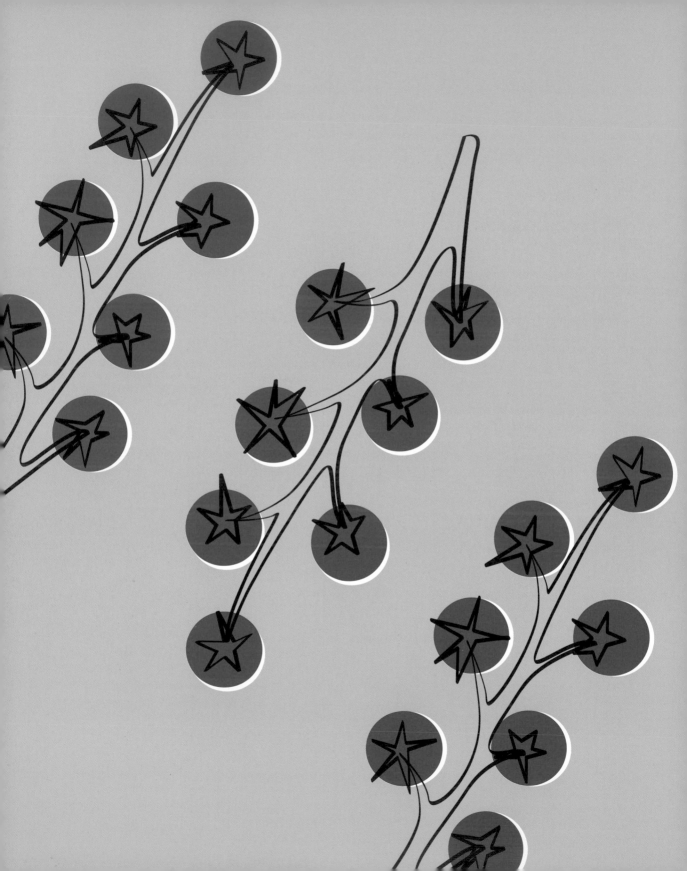

CHAPTER 4

The plant-based benefits

Now we know what the Diversity Diet is, what counts as a healthy plant-based food and the downsides of not adding more plants into your diet. But hey, we're human – which means any change from our norm requires a little extra motivation. And I'm here to give you just that. It's time to ignite your diversity drive by reviewing all the benefits you're likely to experience by embracing those extra plants.

The beauty of focusing on plant-based diversity is that you'll feel benefits immediately, and I've created the recipes in this book to give you all the inspiration and ideas you need to get started. New foods, flavours, textures, colours – I'm talking instant gratification. By eating in this way, you'll start to notice short-term health benefits: better digestion, more energy, less bloating. Before long, the further gains will start to reveal themselves. What's that, you're sleeping better? Your skin's looking good? Fewer aches, pains and seasonal bugs; hormones less haywire? That'll be your well-fed GM returning its thanks! Believe me, I've seen it enough times in clients who've started out sceptical but have increased their plant-based foods and reaped these rewards.

Whatever your current health goals – reducing stress at work, calming tummy troubles, getting to a healthy weight, feeling stronger or more energized, boosting your libido, you name it – the Diversity Diet is likely to help, by nourishing your all-important GM.

Once you understand the power and potential of the gut and how it influences – or even controls – so many systems in our body, I think you'll be on board with its diet and lifestyle preferences. To get there, it helps to think of your GM as a great communicator. It has three distinct ways of speaking to your other organs: via the immune system, the nervous system, and the blood and lymph circulation (that helps get rid of waste and toxins). Let's take a look at some of the pathways that get the most traffic, and you'll start to see just how far-reaching those plant-based benefits can be.

➡ **The gut–brain axis**

➡ **The gut–skin axis**

➡ **The gut–immune axis**

➡ **The gut–hormone axis**

➡ **The gut–metabolism axis**

The gut–brain axis

It's not so hard to imagine a connection between the gut and brain – our digestion and our mental state – if we consider just how many phrases in the English language already exist to describe it. Ever had 'butterflies in your stomach' when nervous? Used your 'gut instinct' to make a difficult decision? Or felt something so deeply it was 'gut-wrenching'?

We've known for over a century that the gut and brain are connected – not just metaphorically but literally, thanks to the impressive web of hundreds of millions of nerves that connect the two, known as the enteric nervous system (ENS). In fact, it's the ENS that originally earned the gut its 'second brain' title because, unlike other organs in the body, the ENS can control the gut independently from our 'primary' brain (aka the central nervous system or CNS). But it's only been in more recent years that the science has uncovered a new key player, and perhaps even the controller, of this intimate relationship: our gut microbiome. And this has become an understandably hot topic.

While research into the role of our GM is still at the new, exciting and so-much-still-to-learn stage, I'm satisfied there's enough evidence from studies conducted on humans to recommend focusing on eating more plants to reduce the risk of, and even help treat, mental health and neurological conditions. Disruption along the gut–brain axis has, for example, been associated with disorders including stress, depression and anxiety, irritable bowel syndrome, autism, schizophrenia, Parkinson's and Alzheimer's diseases. There's even evidence that the state of your GM could be used to predict your risk of depression, persistence of symptoms and how well you recover.

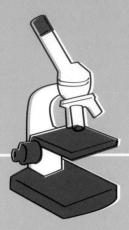

Study snippet

I couldn't talk about the gut–brain axis without sharing one of my favourite scientific studies. If you're not already acquainted, let me introduce you to the 'SMILES' trial – a landmark study investigating whether changing our diets in favour of whole plants could help manage depression. Here is what you need to know:

What they did

People with moderate to severe depression were randomized to receive either befriending therapy (the control group) or a Mediterranean diet full of plant-based diversity for twelve weeks.

The results

Those in the diet group were four times more likely to be in remission (based on clinical questionnaires) after twelve weeks. It's important to note that patients stayed on their antidepressant medication. For me this highlights that diet is best used as an additional or early-stage therapy, so if you are on meds please don't just stop them, but do be reassured that food can really help. Further studies have since reaffirmed this finding – that upping your plants and diversity can have a positive impact on mental health.

Key take-home

Those following the diet full of plant-based foods, including all of the Super Six plant food groups (alongside lean meats, fish, eggs and fermented dairy) – which provided three times more fibre than most of us eat regularly – saw a significant improvement in their mental health. This supports what I regularly see in clinic: whether you have depression or you'd just like to safeguard your emotional state, shifting your diet in favour of whole plants can really help.

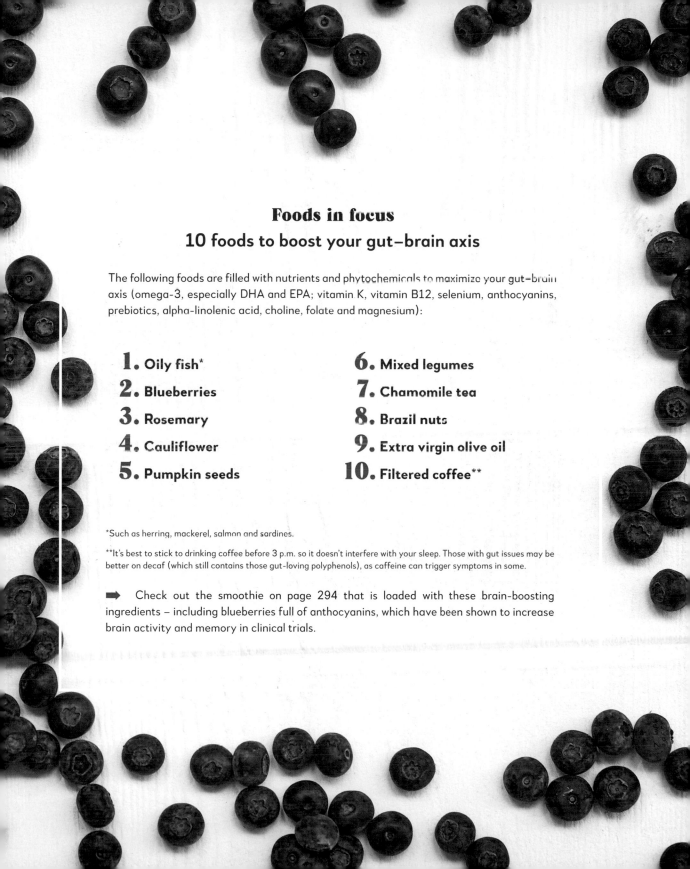

Foods in focus
10 foods to boost your gut–brain axis

The following foods are filled with nutrients and phytochemicals to maximize your gut–brain axis (omega-3, especially DHA and EPA; vitamin K, vitamin B12, selenium, anthocyanins, prebiotics, alpha-linolenic acid, choline, folate and magnesium):

1. Oily fish*
2. Blueberries
3. Rosemary
4. Cauliflower
5. Pumpkin seeds

6. Mixed legumes
7. Chamomile tea
8. Brazil nuts
9. Extra virgin olive oil
10. Filtered coffee**

*Such as herring, mackerel, salmon and sardines.

**It's best to stick to drinking coffee before 3 p.m. so it doesn't interfere with your sleep. Those with gut issues may be better on decaf (which still contains those gut-loving polyphenols), as caffeine can trigger symptoms in some.

➡ Check out the smoothie on page 294 that is loaded with these brain-boosting ingredients – including blueberries full of anthocyanins, which have been shown to increase brain activity and memory in clinical trials.

The gut–skin axis

There's a two-way conversation going on between our microbes and our skin (just like with the brain). And when you think about it, the gut and skin have a lot in common: they're both key players in defending the rest of our body from pathogenic invaders; they house a community of microbes where diversity and stability seem to be important; and they are also in a constant state of renewal, with parts of their linings shedding roughly every week and month, respectively, making them very hungry for nutrition.

What we eat and how we treat our GM often plays out on our skin – as you may have witnessed after a few days of not eating many plant-based foods or having one too many glasses of Prosecco. After all, our skin is an organ that relies on what we feed it to stay alive. One of the earliest observations of this dependency was with scurvy: a doctor in the eighteenth century discovered that citrus fruit (rich in vitamin C) could cure sailors of this disease, one of the first signs of which was skin rashes and bruise-like spots.

Similarly, for skin conditions such as acne, there is a growing body of evidence suggesting that not enough 'healthy' plant-based foods and too many 'unhealthy' plant-based foods like fruit juice, white bread and large amounts of non-fermented dairy (particularly, it seems, skimmed milk) may exacerbate acne through alterations in hormones, among other pathways. That being said, there is no evidence that food alone will cause acne, nor that enjoying these foods in moderation as part of your Diversity Diet will make acne worse. In fact, the stress of aiming for diet 'perfection' in itself can be enough to make your skin break out thanks to the pesky stress hormone, cortisol.

Most of our skin–gut communication happens via the immune system. Simply put, an unbalanced GM (dysbiosis) is thought to set off a response from the immune system, triggering inflammation, which is normally there to protect us from injury or illness. But, like the stress response, inflammation becomes a problem when it's triggered too often and left switched on at a low level over time. Many skin conditions – eczema, rosacea, acne, psoriasis, dermatitis, even premature ageing – are inflammatory in origin, so it figures that a limited GM, lacking in diversity, could be involved.

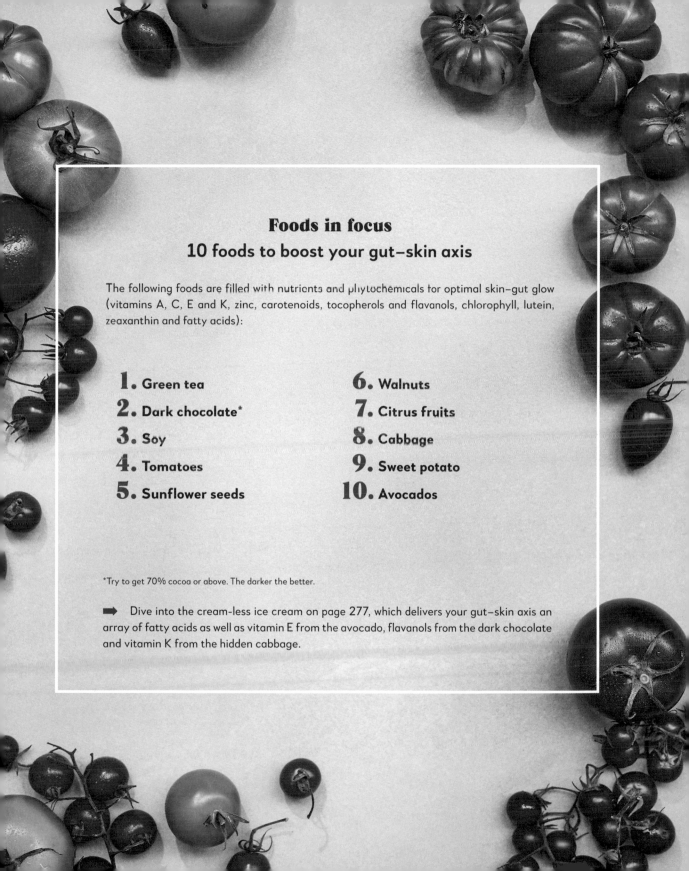

Foods in focus
10 foods to boost your gut–skin axis

The following foods are filled with nutrients and phytochemicals for optimal skin–gut glow (vitamins A, C, E and K, zinc, carotenoids, tocopherols and flavanols, chlorophyll, lutein, zeaxanthin and fatty acids):

1. Green tea
2. Dark chocolate*
3. Soy
4. Tomatoes
5. Sunflower seeds
6. Walnuts
7. Citrus fruits
8. Cabbage
9. Sweet potato
10. Avocados

*Try to get 70% cocoa or above. The darker the better.

➡ Dive into the cream-less ice cream on page 277, which delivers your gut–skin axis an array of fatty acids as well as vitamin E from the avocado, flavanols from the dark chocolate and vitamin K from the hidden cabbage.

If we have a more diverse GM, the microbes keep each other in line and instead can have anti-inflammatory effects. This is partly thanks to the short-chain fatty acids (SCFA) released when they digest fibre, as explained on page 18, which is thought to help our skin counteract some of the environmental damage it faces.

Skin ageing

Even if you don't have any specific skin concerns, it's worth me adding that the gut–skin axis is involved in something we'd all rather slow down: skin ageing. Polyphenols – the beneficial plant chemicals that mostly rely on our GM for absorption in the body (and therefore into the skin) – have also been shown to improve the appearance of ageing. One study using polyphenols from cocoa (hello dark chocolate!) showed reduced facial wrinkles and improved elasticity after twenty-four weeks, compared to placebo (non-polyphenol intervention).

Another study suggested that our skin microbiota can even predict our age, and another found that eating more plants was linked with improved telomere length, a marker of ageing. Now, Botox or that extra portion of vegetables? I'll let you decide . . .

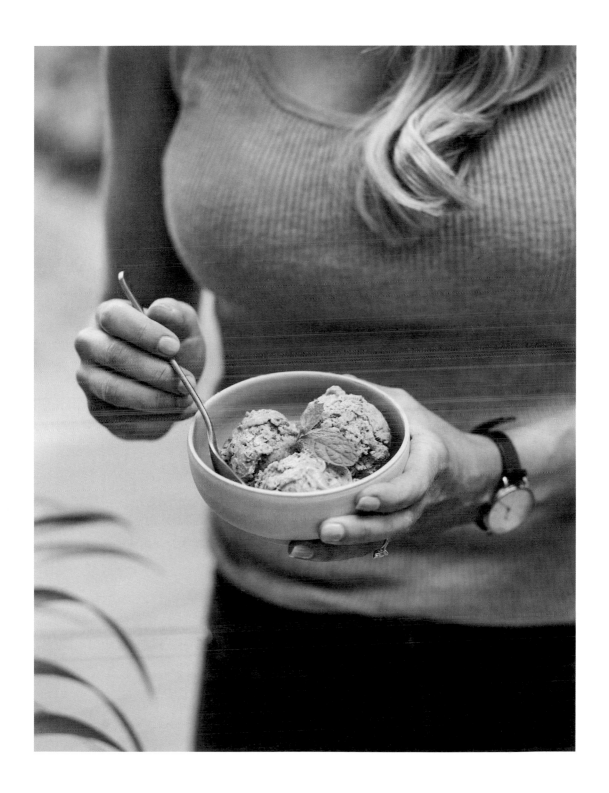

The gut–immune axis

Let's face it, we're all more interested than ever before in bolstering our immunity. Whether it's staving off the common cold and winter flu, protecting ourselves against autoimmune conditions (which are on the rise) or surviving a global pandemic, we want strong defences. 'How can I boost my immunity?' is probably one of the top five questions my clients ask. (Spoiler: we don't actually want 'boosted' immunity; if our immune system is overactive, it can lead to conditions such as autoimmune diseases, as I will explain.)

News headlines are forever proclaiming the next superfood or supplement that's finally going to give us super-immunity. What we don't hear often enough is the fact that immunity is powered by the gut. An impressive 70 per cent of our immune cells actually reside in the gut, alongside our GM. And rather than sitting there rudely ignoring one another, they are in constant communication.

The GM takes on a bit of a parental role, 'training' our immune cells from birth. The microbes teach our immune system what is worth reacting to (like disease-causing microbes) and what is safe (like proteins found in certain foods). Without our GM, our immunity would be pretty inefficient – think amateur athlete versus elite athlete (I know who I'd rather have on my side).

So, one of the best ways we can support our immunity is by supporting our GM – keeping it healthy by keeping our diet diverse and plant-based. The alternative? A likely disturbed GM and a poorly trained immune system that overreacts to innocent bystanders (cue allergies and autoimmune conditions) and underreacts to the real culprits (giving a free pass to cold- and flu-causing viruses).

Autoimmune conditions

There are more than eighty different autoimmune conditions (where the immune system turns on itself) and, although we still have a lot to learn, there seem to be three main factors – keys to turn the autoimmune lock – that determine whether you fall into the 5–8 per cent of people diagnosed with one:

1. **Genetics** (we can't change these – thanks, Mum and Dad)

---

2. **Our environment** (where we live, pollution, lifestyle)

---

3. **Our GM** (the newly recognized player)

Our understanding of the exact role of our GM is still in its infancy, but the research is fascinating. A reduced GM diversity has been observed in a series of autoimmune conditions, as we touched on earlier, but this type of research only demonstrates that there's an association between the two, rather than one causing the other.

The first real clue that a dysbiotic GM plays a causal role in autoimmune responses was originally found in mice studies. Microbe-free mice (born into a sterile environment, so they have no GM) have been demonstrated to be protected against developing autoimmune conditions. Subsequent studies showed that transplanting the dysbiotic GM from people with autoimmune conditions into healthy mice (yes, a poop transplant, aka faecal microbiota transplant or FMT) could trigger autoimmunity, where the immune system turns on itself.

This finding has been translated into early-stage human studies, which have indicated that, in some people, FMT could be used to reverse ulcerative colitis, a type of inflammatory bowel disease that involves autoimmune activation – watch this space.

Viral defence

In terms of defence against viruses, there's pretty convincing evidence that altering our GM increases our resistance, particularly when it comes to the common cold and flu (acute URTIs, or upper respiratory tract infections). In 2015, a review was conducted by a global independent network of researchers known as Cochrane, looking at all clinical trials on probiotics for acute URTIs. They found that specific probiotics could reduce the number of people getting a URTI by 47 per cent, as well as reducing the duration of an episode by nearly two days if they did get it, compared to placebo. This indicates that, by giving your GM a boost, you boost your cold and flu resistance too.

And what about *that* virus? If ever there were proof we're living in a microbial world – inside and out – it came in the form of COVID-19. Research has shown some people with the virus had decreased levels of beneficial bacteria – and that their GM could predict who was more likely to become severely unwell with COVID-19. Another small initial study showed that a specific multi-strain probiotic (when added to standard medical therapy) reduced people's risk of developing respiratory failure, compared to those who just received standard therapy. Now, it's very early days and this particular probiotic isn't commercially available yet – but fingers crossed that changes as evidence mounts!

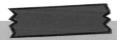

Case study

When the World Health Organization declared a public health emergency at the end of January 2020, the severity of the new coronavirus became crystal clear. With my husband, Thomas, working on the frontline as an NHS GP, I knew he was incredibly vulnerable and I wanted to do everything I could to help support his immune system. So, I took a deep dive into the scientific literature and emerged a week later with a plan – which, as you may expect after reading this section, was no different to the advice I give in this book . . . reaffirming that what's good for the gut is good for the immune system – they really do go hand in hand.

We were both working pretty crazy hours, so I made sure the plan was as easy as possible to implement. I focused on simple but effective evidence-based actions that we could keep up for the long haul. We enjoyed quick and simple plant-powered and fibre-filled meals (which formed the basis of the Busy People menu plan on pages 124–125), committed to being asleep by 10 p.m. each night, as well as setting aside 5 minutes every evening to destress and reconnect, using many of the strategies outlined on page 116.

Fast forward four months to when the antibody tests became available to the frontline healthcare workers: we discovered that Thomas had actually contracted COVID-19. Yet he never showed one single symptom. He even commented that, despite the intensity of everything, he felt better than ever within himself. While he was somewhat surprised, I knew the plan was grounded in science. Now, it's important to remember that this is just anecdotal evidence and is of course no guarantee, but it does support the studies so far that nourishing your gut may very well reduce your risk of becoming unwell if you do contract COVID-19.

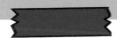

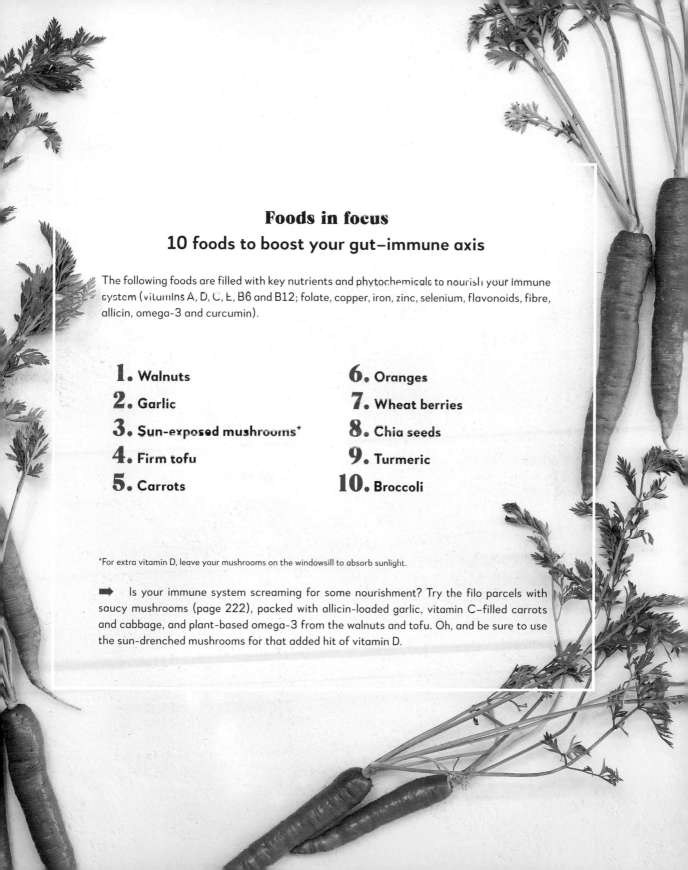

Foods in focus
10 foods to boost your gut–immune axis

The following foods are filled with key nutrients and phytochemicals to nourish your immune system (vitamins A, D, C, E, B6 and B12; folate, copper, iron, zinc, selenium, flavonoids, fibre, allicin, omega-3 and curcumin).

1. Walnuts
2. Garlic
3. Sun-exposed mushrooms*
4. Firm tofu
5. Carrots

6. Oranges
7. Wheat berries
8. Chia seeds
9. Turmeric
10. Broccoli

*For extra vitamin D, leave your mushrooms on the windowsill to absorb sunlight.

➡ Is your immune system screaming for some nourishment? Try the filo parcels with saucy mushrooms (page 222), packed with allicin-loaded garlic, vitamin C–filled carrots and cabbage, and plant-based omega-3 from the walnuts and tofu. Oh, and be sure to use the sun-drenched mushrooms for that added hit of vitamin D.

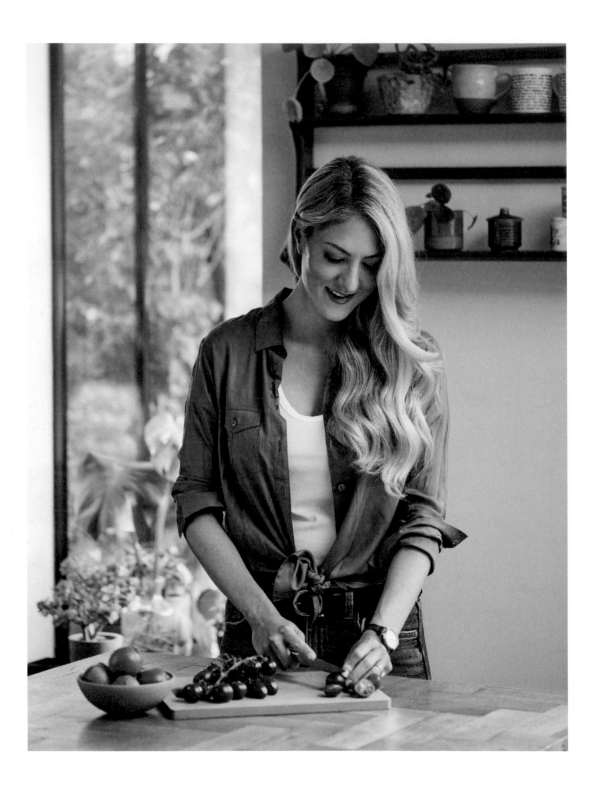

The gut–hormone axis

Yet another role your all-powerful gut plays: it makes and regulates hormones. From thyroid hormones to appetite and sex hormones, our GM is proving to be quite the hormone dispenser. For a quick and clear example, remember those microbe-free mice? A study found they had abnormal sexual development and growth-hormone secretion, with fewer gender differences. Essentially, the male mice became feminized and vice versa – all because they lacked a GM to produce and help regulate their hormones.

These findings have fuelled my interest in whether harnessing the power of our GM can perhaps help us better navigate the hormonal rollercoaster that is being female. Don't worry, guys, this area is not exclusive to women; not only does oestrogen affect you too, a number of our gut microbes are able to produce testosterone and there are several parallels with oestrogen balance – the clinical research just needs to catch up.

Oestrogen balance

Oestrogen is known us a key female hormone because it controls our reproductive cycle from puberty to menopause – as well as each menstrual cycle. It also plays a role in the health of our heart and blood vessels, bones, breasts, skin, hair and even our brain.

Our GM is able to influence circulating oestrogen levels thanks to an enzyme it produces called beta-glucuronidase, which can turn inactive oestrogen into active oestrogen, recycling it from our gut back into our circulation. As a result, GM dysbiosis has been shown to negatively impact circulating oestrogen levels, which can play a role in common hormonal conditions ranging from polycystic ovary syndrome, endometriosis and infertility to breast cancer.

Equally, an abundant and diverse GM is more likely to keep oestrogen levels balanced, with the potential to reduce menopausal symptoms and conditions caused by imbalances in oestrogen levels. This may very well explain why in a one-year intervention study of over 17,000 menopausal women, those eating more fibre – including vegetables, fruit and soy – experienced a 19 per cent reduction in hot flushes compared to the control group.

And one systematic review (where they pool together individual trials on a topic) found that supplementing a healthy diet with specific probiotics could improve several blood markers of polycystic ovary syndrome, including hormones, compared to controls.

Insulin

It's not just about sexual health – there are hormones that control appetite, metabolism (more on those on page 74) and the hormone that regulates our blood sugars, insulin. Maintaining a healthy gut has been linked to a reduced risk of metabolic syndrome (a combination of elevated blood sugars, blood pressure and body weight) – which, if not managed, can develop into type 2 diabetes. One very small but landmark study showed that transplanting the gut microbes from healthy, lean people (aka poop donors) into people with metabolic syndrome, was able to improve insulin sensitivity, i.e. improve their health markers. But, in case you are tempted by FMT, I must emphasize that this is only early days, and outside of treating life-threatening gut infections, FMT is not yet ready for practice given the associated risks, such as incidentally transplanting conditions like depression (as shown in mice studies). That being said, all of this research does support the role of nourishing our GM through diet and lifestyle to help in the management (and prevention) of a wide range of disease.

We still have so much to learn, and while it's very unlikely to be solely down to our GM, I think it's fair to say that, for hormonal balance, you're going to want to keep your GM onside.

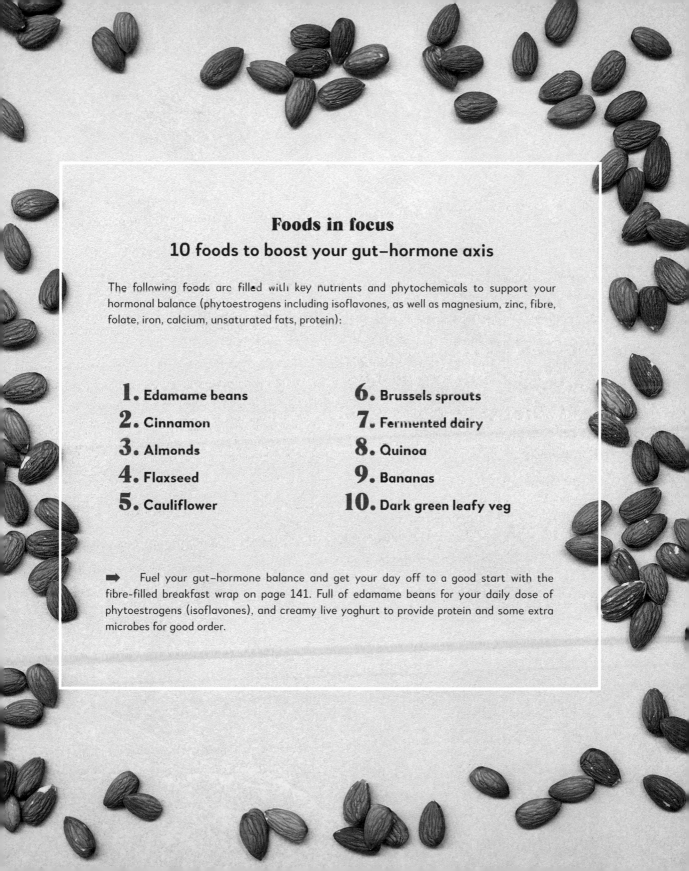

Foods in focus
10 foods to boost your gut–hormone axis

The following foods are filled with key nutrients and phytochemicals to support your hormonal balance (phytoestrogens including isoflavones, as well as magnesium, zinc, fibre, folate, iron, calcium, unsaturated fats, protein):

1. Edamame beans
2. Cinnamon
3. Almonds
4. Flaxseed
5. Cauliflower
6. Brussels sprouts
7. Fermented dairy
8. Quinoa
9. Bananas
10. Dark green leafy veg

➡ Fuel your gut–hormone balance and get your day off to a good start with the fibre-filled breakfast wrap on page 141. Full of edamame beans for your daily dose of phytoestrogens (isoflavones), and creamy live yoghurt to provide protein and some extra microbes for good order.

The gut–metabolism axis

We're all aware of the link between what we eat and whether we lose, gain or maintain weight. In fact, for many people, that link can become all-consuming (if you'll pardon the pun), taking all the pleasure out of eating as we struggle to balance cravings with what we think we 'should' be eating. But here's some news I think you're going to like . . .

Forget calories in and out (more of that in chapter 5) or restrictive diets that are low fat, low carb and so on. There's a definite link between our GM and our metabolism, and we can use this in our favour.

Our gut microbes and the chemicals they make when they digest the fibre we eat from plants can impact appetite. These chemicals, such as SCFA, essentially tell our body we've had enough. In turn, this halts the production of hunger hormones such as ghrelin, and increases the 'I'm full' hormones such as leptin. This likely explains why it's often fibre intake, independent of calorie intake or type of diet, that results in healthier weight and greater dietary adherence – as shown in the appropriately named 2019 POUNDS study.

And it's not just SCFA that do the 'food ordering'; other chemicals produced by our GM are thought to target the reward network part of the brain, which influence our relationship with food and our tendency towards emotional eating.

Weight management

Our GM is involved in energy harvesting. Our microbes scavenge for undigested food and turn it into energy – which can be stored as fat if it's not used. But different microbes are better than others at energy harvesting and our GMs are all completely unique, which could explain why some people seem to be able to graze all day, while others feel like they just have to look at a plate to put on weight.

The gut–metabolism axis doesn't stop there. Microbes and their metabolites have been linked with 'turning on' genes in your body that are related to fat distribution. They can also affect glucose and fat production and storage in the liver. Added to the fact that our microbes may influence our taste receptors and mood, it becomes pretty clear that having a higher body weight is way more complex than simply eating too much and not exercising enough. Your microbiome plays a starring role – and hey, by the end of all this research we'll probably find it's an Oscar-winning director!

If you are feeling a little defeated by these findings, remember the empowering truth of it all – much of our GM is in our control, dictated by how we feed and treat it. In fact, several studies, albeit in animals, have shown that polyphenols (those plant chemicals with antioxidant powers) found in a wide range of fruit and veg play a prominent role in preventing weight gain by increasing metabolic rate. This mechanism appears to translate in human studies too, where those who eat more plants tend to also have a lower body weight.

In a nutshell, feed your GM well and it's likely to keep everything else in check. So step off the scales, put down the calorie-counting calculator and just eat more plants! That's what I advised my client Jackie, and it worked . . .

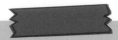

Case study

Aged fifty-two, Jackie was going through menopause and had been dieting on and off for years – observing that this behaviour was now impacting her daughter's relationship with food too. When a routine blood test found she had pre-diabetes, Jackie knew she had to do something.

I worked with her over four months, introducing small, practical changes. She quit calorie counting, dropped the sweeteners that were making her crave and binge on foods high in added sugar, and shifted to the Diversity Diet.

The latter was tricky, as Jackie's years of dieting had given her an aversion to vegetables – she associated them with boring, restricted eating. I jumped at the chance to demonstrate the Diversity Diet was anything but! Simple tricks like making batches of roast veg with extra virgin olive oil, smoked paprika and rock salt (instead of her usual boiled and bland veg) soon convinced all the family that plants could be tasty.

I encouraged Jackie to add extra veg to every meal and mix up her go-to pasta or rice with minimally processed wholegrains such as quinoa, freekeh and wheat berries – which she was surprised to find were actually stocked in her local supermarket – and she quickly admitted to loving these new textures and flavours. (Not sure what these wholegrains are? Check out pages 102–103).

I showed Jackie how easy it was to add plant-based foods to regular meals, like lentils to lasagne (see the hearty lasagne on page 237) and quinoa to burgers (check out the smoky beet burger on page 213) and naturally cutting back on meat as a result. The thing that really drove Jackie to making these long-term changes was that these were meals all the family would enjoy and benefit from, at no extra expense (in fact, there was a cost saving with reduced meat!).

We also worked on her phobia of fat, introducing healthy, filling options like full-fat live yoghurt and whole nuts. And I showed Jackie mindfulness techniques like the one on page 111, which resulted in her feeling more satisfied after each meal and so less likely to overeat.

Four months on? Her weight was down and she was fitting into those jeans that used to stare at her from the back of the wardrobe. What's more, blood tests revealed she no longer had pre-diabetes – reflecting the scientific evidence that you really can reverse many of these chronic conditions through diet. Jackie reported that her hot flushes had reduced, she felt less irritable and her skin felt more hydrated. Oh, and her whole family powered through flu season, symptom-free.

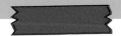

Foods in focus
10 foods to boost your gut—metabolism axis

The following foods are filled with key nutrients and phytochemicals to support your hungry GM (fibre, including resistant starch, beta-glucan and prebiotics; polyphenols, calcium, capsaicin, acetic acid, live microbes, iodine, protein):

1. Natural live yoghurt
2. Jumbo oats
3. Balsamic vinegar
4. Butter beans
5. Ginger

6. Fennel
7. Cold potato salad
8. Pistachios
9. Chilli peppers
10. Grapefruit

➡ Fuel your metabolism with the smoked mackerel, new potato and apple salad on page 195, giving you plenty of resistant starch from the cooked and cooled potatoes, vinegar from the mustard, fermented dairy in the dressing, polyphenols from the fennel bulbs, and iodine and protein from the mackerel.

The take home

There is a lot to digest (sorry, *take in*) in this chapter. But I didn't want to skim over it. And that's because I'm passionate about communicating the far-reaching benefits of improving your gut health by going plant-based. As I hope I've demonstrated here, the Diversity Diet isn't only about better digestion. It's not even just about your long-term reduced risk of many (so many!) health conditions. It's about nurturing a system of communication that affects every aspect of your health. Who knew it was so easy to make such a big impact?

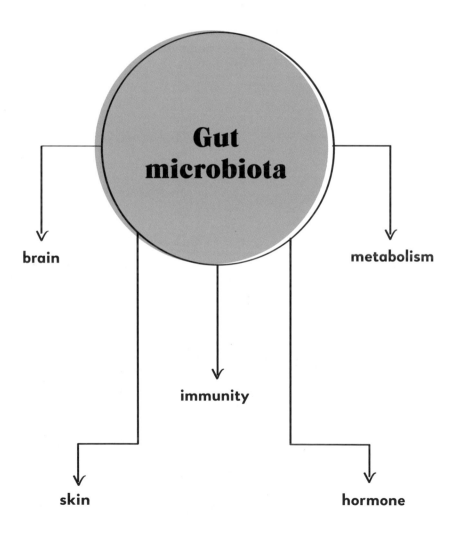

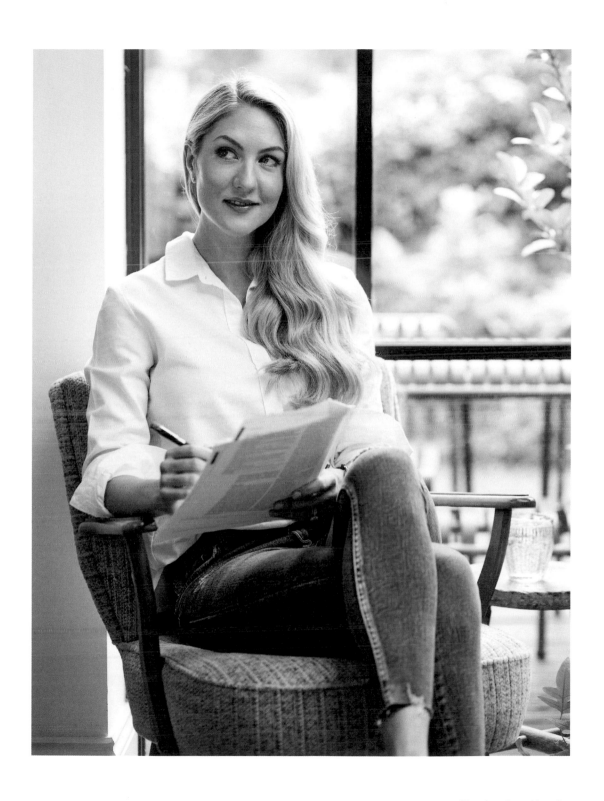

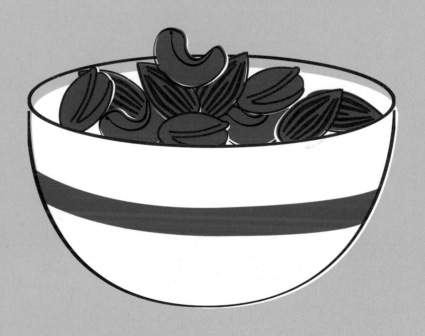

CHAPTER 5

What's holding you back?

Now, of course, I'm hoping you don't see any barriers to the Diversity Diet and that you're already flicking forward to the recipes, raring to get going. But if we're going to do this together, the right way, for the long term, let's really do it and leave no doubt in your mind, no lingering hang-ups, no secret allegiance to past food fads.

In this chapter, I'm going to run through some common misconceptions about going plant-based. These are some questions I often get asked by my clients, but they're easily answered. It's time to bust some myths!

If I don't count calories, surely I'll gain weight?

Ah, the great calorie conundrum. This one is a biggie, I get that. If you've grown up with more than a passing interest in food, weight loss and eating healthily, you might have fallen into the calorie-counting trap. It's hard not to, when the idea of balancing calories eaten versus calories burned is still the basis of most diet plans, government guidance and even medical professionals' advice when it comes to losing weight. So why would you suddenly forget about calories and start gorging on plants?

I hear you. And I'm going to explain why I've designed the menu plans and recipes without any mention of those pesky Cs.

1. **What's listed on the packet, or on your food-tracking app, or online somewhere, is not as accurate as you've been led to believe.** That's because a food's calorie count is typically determined in the laboratory, simply by burning the whole food and extracting every last calorie from it. And that process is very different from what actually happens to it in our intricate digestive systems. Take almonds, for example. Human digestion studies have shown that they provide 30 per cent fewer calories than what's labelled on the pack. You see, unlike in the laboratory studies, humans (and our gut microbes) don't extract every last calorie from whole plant foods. With highly processed foods, on the other hand, most of the 'digesting' has already been done for us by big machines, making the calories much more accessible.

2. **Food has what's called a thermogenic effect.** That's when your body burns calories while eating and digesting. This is another reason all calories (as labelled) are not 'equal', so to speak, because your body's processing will counter some of them – and here's the important bit – depending on the *specific* food. Whole foods like fruit, veg and nuts that need chewing, breaking down and more digesting have a higher thermogenic effect than ultra-processed foods.

    One study in particular found that the calories burned digesting a meal consisting of processed foods were around 50 per cent lower than those burned after a whole-food meal, despite both containing the same total carbs, fat and protein. It might not sound enough to make a lot of difference, but over a month, a year, a lifetime? It certainly adds up.

Further research in 2019 found that people told to eat as much as they liked gained significantly more weight when given ultra-processed foods than when given unprocessed options, again even when the meals were matched for carbs, fat and protein. This validates what I have witnessed over the past decade working with clients: that switching from processed to whole foods is a better weight-management strategy than counting 'calories in'.

These sorts of findings are reiterated time and time again in research and explain why we often experience a lack of satiety (that lasting feeling of fullness) after eating processed foods. You've been there, I'm sure – enjoyed a fast-food meal, felt absolutely stuffed, then weirdly open to round two an hour later?

If a food has already been broken down for you, your body has less work to do and it's less satisfying. An apple takes longer to eat and is way more filling than apple sauce, which itself is more satiating than a glass of apple juice. And that's because a whole apple contains fibre and water bound up in what we call a 'food matrix'. The more manufacturers break a food down, often the more fibre they lose – along with that all-important food matrix

So, if you want to feel fuller for longer and more satisfied after a meal, opt for a piece of fruit rather than a glass of juice, or jumbo oats not refined porridge quick oats – think whole plants that have been minimally 'tampered' with. By understanding this and knowing why this advice really works, it makes those simple changes much more appealing.

Food is way more than just calories

As we saw in chapter 2, plant-based foods are packed with thousands of different nutrients and phytochemicals. Sure, a KitKat and a banana might contain similar calories – and your food-tracking app won't treat them any differently. But your body will! It'll make great use of the banana's potassium to support healthy blood pressure. Your GM will feast on the banana's prebiotic fibre. And your whole being may even get a kick from its serotonin (which you may know as the 'happy hormone').

Tip
Ditch the calorie fixation. Not only are the calorie labels inaccurate (our digestive systems are more intricate than that!) but eating whole plant foods has been shown to help with weight management, without restricting calories.

Food is also about culture, nostalgia and family memories. It's sociable and enjoyable. I'm not about to destroy all that by asking you to put numbers on everything. That, to me, is a recipe for healthy-eating hell.

By eating a plant-based diet we tend to feel more connected to nature and the world around us. As hippie-dippie as that sounds, the research shows this really does put us back in touch with real flavours and textures, and it's why seasonal eating has become such a trend in recent years.

If you're still not convinced that there's no need to fixate on calories when upping your plant intake, and if weight management is your main concern when thinking about how to improve your diet, here's something that is sure to put those thoughts to bed. A meta-analysis (where researchers pull together the results of individual studies, 15 in this case) has shown that plant-based eating can result in a significant reduction in body weight, without any restrictions on portion size or calorie intake. The proof is in the pudding.

But I'll definitely put on weight if I gorge on nuts and avocado . . .

There are certain foods I call 'halo foods' because they've hit the headlines for being healthy and now are everywhere – recipes, cafés, all over Instagram – to signal that people are making 'good' food choices. Indeed, they *are* good for us, but that doesn't mean we should eat them to excess and to the exclusion of other plants.

Peanut butter, I'm looking at you. Yes, you're damn tasty. Yes, you're a valuable source of plant protein, healthy fats, vitamins and minerals, and a decent slow-release source of energy. But you're not the only healthy plant food out there.

Another huge one is smashed avocado. I'm on to you too. I know you're a good source of unsaturated fat, fibre, potassium and folate – but you're not the only one. There are plenty more healthy foods not getting a look-in thanks to you hogging the limelight.

It all comes back to the D-word: *diversity*. Sure, have your PB and avo, but mix it up. Get those plant points to 30 and beyond (including a portion of nuts or seeds each day, see page 17).

If you do find yourself feeling 'out of control' and eating one plant-based food or group much more than any other (which can be quite common in those coming from a restrictive diet), it is worth exploring the mindful-eating exercise on page 111. It's all about getting you back in tune with your body's hunger and satiety signals.

Won't I be protein-deficient if I only eat plants?

First, let's recap chapter 1. This is about being plant-*based* not plants-*only*. Animal produce, if you want it, is definitely still on the menu. Vegetarians, famously, have a reduced risk of all-cause mortality (death for any reason), but studies also show the same is true of diets that simply place more of an emphasis on plants.

Second, plants contain protein too. I'm going to say the D-word again, because so long as your focus is on *diversity*, you'll likely be getting all the protein building blocks (amino acids) you need. And if you're talking about building your muscle mass to achieve a fitness goal, an increasing number of professional athletes are vegan, reaffirming that protein from plants is more than sufficient in supporting our bodies when training. For more on this, flick back to page 39.

I'm vegan, so I'm there already, right?

You'd be forgiven for thinking that you've already ticked all the healthy boxes by following a vegan diet, but the truth is that simply excluding animal products isn't what will support your GM and therefore your overall health. Instead, you need to look at what sort of plant-based foods your vegan diet is made up of. Remember that plant-based diet index on page 30? The key is how processed and diverse your plants are.

As vegan diets have moved into the mainstream, food manufacturers have responded by making more and more convenience foods for 'vegans on the go'. I'm talking fake ham, fake frankfurters, meatless sausage rolls, vegan 'cheese', you name it. While this might seem like progress, these kinds of ultra-processed food are not what your GM needs. Soy protein, in particular, is used to make many meat-substitute products. But to get to that malleable product with a meaty texture, it has been through lots of processes since its original life as whole soybeans – not to mention the food additives, several of which are currently under investigation as GM disruptors. These sorts of foods are also often high in salt (which, in excess, can negatively impact our GM).

So, although you might be following a vegan diet and feel pretty healthy in that decision, highly processed meat alternatives are definitely not doing as much for you as their whole-food counterparts.

What you *can't* get from plants

While we can get a huge amount of the nutrients we need from eating plants, going vegan can make it a little more challenging to meet your body's needs for specific things. This is because animal foods are the main and often most easily absorbed source of several of the essential nutrients, including calcium, iron, zinc, vitamin B12, iodine, selenium, choline and long-chain omega-3 fatty acids (DHA and EPA).

This is why I generally recommend a plant-*based* diet rather than an exclusively vegan diet. But if you do want to take the exclusive approach, by all means go ahead. I generally recommend my vegan clients supplement their diet with B12 (at least 10 micrograms a day) and algae-derived DHA and EPA fatty acids (around 250 milligrams a day), as well as making a concerted effort to get those missing nutrients from foods like nutritional yeast, fortified plant-based milks, Brazil nuts, nori, walnuts, flaxseed and seeded sourdough.

Interestingly, our GM actually can make its own B12. This is why there is a subset of vegans who don't need to take supplements. However, most GMs in the Western world don't make enough, so in my opinion it's best to be safe and up your intake if you don't have access to testing.

Plant-based food is too expensive and hard to get hold of

I'm not denying that there are plenty of overpriced plant-based stores and delis where a week's shopping could cost you a month's wages. But despite what they'd love you to believe, you certainly don't need to shop in those places to follow the Diversity Diet. Everything in this book is available from your mainstream supermarket of choice, your local greengrocer or farmers' market, or your corner shop; and lots of it you can even grow on a veg patch or allotment. Sure, you may want to branch out and experiment with exotic fruit and veg or exciting plant-based condiments, and they may take a little hunting for (although is there anything you can't get online these days?). But the bottom line is plant-based diversity can be easy *and* affordable – just stick to my four tips on page 89. Not only have they helped many of my patients on a budget, but they are what I lived by when I moved to London and struggled to make ends meet.

You don't need to take my word for it either. A study looking at the costs of going plant-based showed that, despite the participants' initial perception, the cost of their weekly grocery basket actually went down over time.

Cost-saving tips

1. Buy fruit and vegetables in season.

The recipes in this book are very much adaptable by season. If it says pomegranate (winter fruit) but you're making it in summer, go with strawberries instead – you can't really go wrong. How do you know which fruit and vegetables are in season? The price! They're around half the price when in season. You can also check out the seasonality lists on my website thequthealthdoctor.com.

2. Bulk out your meat dishes with legumes.

The ultimate cost-saver, whether you soak and cook them from scratch or opt for the tins. Even the more 'fancy' protein options such as tofu are cheaper than meat.

3. Don't let fruit and veg go off!

Many of the recipes in this book are labelled with a 'fridge raid' icon (see page 118). This is your opportunity to use up any wilting veg or bruised fruit. And don't forget about the freezer. If you buy in bulk, particularly plants in season, utilize the freezer as your ultimate preserver. For most vegetables, just blanch them in boiling water for a few minutes before chilling and freezing. Fruit, on the other hand, is ready to go straight in! The exception being fruit and veg with high water content, like watermelon and cucumber. These are best eaten fresh.

4. Take your own snacks when out and about.

This means that you don't have to succumb to the £3 'vegan' energy balls when hunger strikes. I've got a recipe on page 142 that costs less than 20p per ball to make, and you can keep them in the freezer for months.

I can get all the nutrients I need – without all the cooking – by taking supplements

I'm afraid I hear this a lot, but it isn't entirely true. You remember Harry from chapter 2, who thought he could hit his daily plant quota with his meal-replacement shakes? It didn't work for him and it's unlikely to work for you. These shakes claim to provide all the fat, carbs, protein, vitamins and minerals you need each day. But as you know by now, real food offers so much more nutrition, not to mention flavour (and where's that all-important food matrix in liquid food?). So, let Silicon Valley supply your tech, not your nutrition.

Dietary supplements are big business. From single vitamins and minerals to multi-formulations and blends for specific purposes (brain power, digestion, sleep), you can buy them all in capsule form. And sometimes, undoubtedly, they're helpful. Vitamin D, for example, is a must for everyone living in countries with limited sunlight exposure during the winter months, and there are several cases where I recommend specific supplements (such as probiotics, fibre supplements and peppermint capsules) in my clinic. But these really are on a case-by-case basis, and the formulations are backed by clinical trials. The chances are you don't need most, if any, of those bottles of vitamins that line the shelves of high-street pharmacies, no matter how convincing their 'boost your energy' and 'strengthen your nails' claims are.

Not only can they be a waste of money, we also know that some isolated nutrients can be harmful in high doses or can interact with other medications (one example is vitamin E). If you take a range of formulations and don't study all the labels closely, you could easily be taking too much of certain vitamins or minerals. On the other hand, it's hard to overdose on single nutrients the way Mother Nature packages them. Food contains what you need, in safe portions, which is why eating a diverse diet is the most effective and fail-safe way to give your body what it needs.

Will I have to give up my favourite foods?

This is not an all-or-nothing approach. I said it right at the start – it's about enriching, not restricting. I don't want anyone to give up something they love. There's no way I'm going to live my best life without having white chocolate!

That's the beauty of the Diversity Diet: it's about 'adding in' plants for your microbes to enjoy, alongside your taste buds' favourites, which is why I designed my crave-busting pistachio berry bursts (page 282).

Rather than giving up and feeling deprived, you'll soon find that by adding in plants you'll discover new flavours and recipes that will have your taste buds wishing you'd started this way of eating much earlier. Many of the recipes in this book will become your new favourites – and because they're so filling you'll naturally feel more satisfied, with fewer cravings.

The earlier you start with children the better too, so be sure to give my menu plan for all the family a try (see page 122) and you'll have the kids on board before you know it. But rest assured, there's always room for your old recipe favourites, and you may even be enticed to make a few tweaks after reading chapter 6. Plant-based is tasty and fun!

Bloating, cramps . . . wind! I'm sorry, but too much of the plant stuff just doesn't agree with me

This is a really important conversation to have, because all too often I see people in clinic who have experienced such severe gut symptoms that they have stripped most of the fibre out of their diet – and are frightened about adding it back in. One of the most common questions I get asked is: 'Why can I tolerate meat, fish and refined carbs like white rice, but not veg or wholegrains?'

The simple answer is these foods, unlike high-fibre foods such as veg, are mostly digested by human enzymes higher up in your gut. They don't rely on your GM to digest them. For the 'smooth' (symptomless) digestion of fibre, however, you need two things:

1. **Microbes that are equipped with enough enzymes to digest the fibre you're eating.**
If over a short period of time you go from a very low-fibre diet to one that has loads of fibre, your digestion is unlikely to feel smooth – most people can expect bloating, a change in pooping habits and so on, as the body adjusts. As we discussed in chapter 3, this is partly because your microbe profile hasn't yet adapted to reflect the foods you're giving it (picture a new café opening that is overwhelmed by the demand in its first few weeks, but then hires more staff to handle all the customers). It's also worth keeping in mind that a little gas and bloating is the sign of a well-fed GM, i.e. it's completely normal and isn't to be feared.

Try this: A slow introduction of plant diversity, to give your microbes time to assemble all the right 'tools' to get to work on that great fibre. That could mean starting by adding half a 'normal' portion of plants per day. Try half a piece of fruit, or ¼ cup of legumes per sitting, or stick to just one of the high-fibre recipes in this book per day. For others with more sensitive guts, you might want to start with a quarter of a portion and work up to half and then a whole portion over several months. For more tips turn to page 114.

2. **A relaxed gut.**
If you have an uptight gut – meaning you're stressed (which can be unconscious for some), or perhaps your gut itself is stressed following an infection (food poisoning, gastritis, etc.) – your gut wall is not very efficient at absorbing the gas and other chemicals that are produced by your GM during fibre digestion. Instead of the gas being efficiently absorbed across your gut wall and into your bloodstream (where it's then breathed out through your lungs), it can get trapped in your gut, causing those symptoms of bloating, cramps, etc. This can explain why some days you're fine with a specific higher-fibre food, but other days it feels like a total disaster . . . The annoying truth is, it's not always about the food, but the state of your gut–brain axis.

Try this: Alongside the slow fibre introduction described above, find time to de-stress with some yoga, mindfulness or whatever else brings your mind and body into a relaxed state. The science shows it really can help your digestion. For more tips on this, turn to pages 111–112.

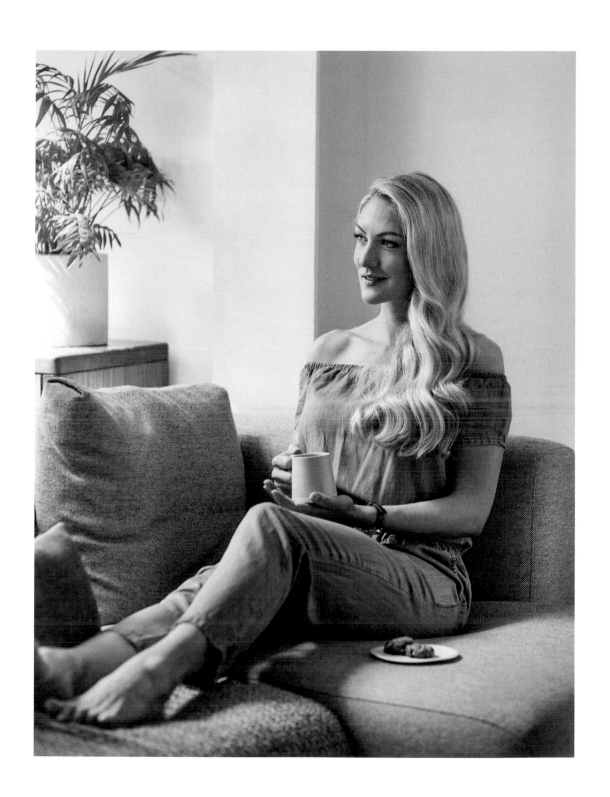

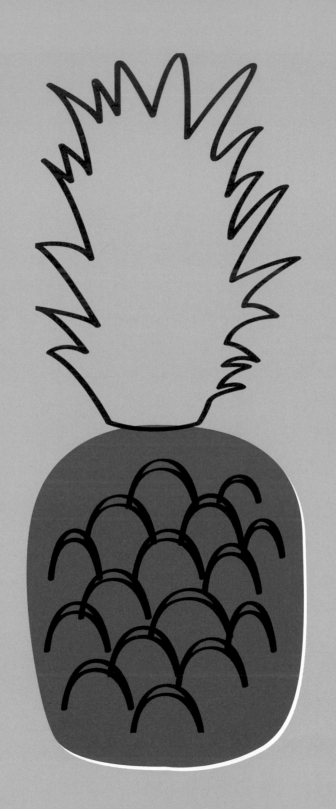

CHAPTER 6

The Diversity Diet toolkit

Ready to get going? I hope by now you're at least tempted to join the Diversity Diet revolution. The next (and final) step is to show you that making the transition is easy – and dare I say even a little exciting – as we take your taste buds on a culinary adventure. Sure, knowledge is key, and understanding why you're making a change will underpin your motivation and commitment. But I'm also a big believer in practical advice. It's about that extra helping hand to make the transition to a more nutritious and delicious way of eating that's full of a variety of plants. Think of this chapter as your Diversity Diet toolkit.

My top diversity hacks

Looking for easy ways to get your weekly plant points to 30 and beyond? Why not give one of these **quick switches**, **habit formers** and **easy adds** a try each week?

Quick switches:

1. Peckish? Swap crisps for a handful of toasted nuts or seeds, or try saving your potato or butternut squash peelings to roast in the oven for a crispy snack (see my sweet potato gnocchi recipe on page 244). A great way to reduce your food waste too!

2. If you're making a fruit crumble, substitute a third of the flour with oats and another third with ground almonds (check out page 285 for my gut-loving version).

3. Don't just add kidney beans to your chilli; replace with mixed beans for greater diversity.

4. Switch your single piece of fruit for half a cup of mixed berries (fresh or frozen).

5. Fancy crackers and dip? Sub out those plain boring crackers for a seedy selection (check out my recipes on page 175) or veg sticks such as green beans, sugar snap peas and asparagus - no chopping necessary!

Habit formers:

1. Every time you go to serve up a meal at home, stop and think, 'What could I add?' Chop a banana over your muesli (see page 143 for my DIY plant-packed muesli), add some sprouts to your sandwich, slice a tomato on to your plate – every bit counts.

2. Are you a habit shopper? We all do it! Once a month, allow an extra thirty minutes in the supermarket to browse the plant-food aisles. You may be surprised by the different varieties on offer. Or seek out a new farmers' market or farm shop to visit, to give you some inspiration.

3. Stock up on frozen veg and fruit – so when you've got nothing fresh left, it doesn't matter. For extra diversity, buy mixed bags of both.

4. Whether you're eating out or cooking at home, aim to try a different cuisine once a week – it'll introduce you to new plants and flavours.

5. Consider signing up for a local farm or veg-box delivery if you have access to one, as each delivery gives you different plants and encourages you to try new things.

Easy adds:

1. Most, if not all, dishes will benefit from the addition of some herbs or spices, which also add some extra phytochemicals to your meal. Keep your dried herb and spice jars out where you can see them, so you don't forget to sprinkle a few into each meal.

2. No casserole, stew, risotto or pie is complete without one more vegetable than the recipe says – it can be as simple as adding a tin of lentils or chickpeas (think of the cost saving too; it'll go twice as far).

3. Make up a seed shaker and add a sprinkle to cereals, yoghurt, smoothies and salads. Seeds work as a tasty, crunchy topper for scrambled eggs, avocado on toast, or soup.

4. Grow your own fresh herbs you only need a windowsill – and add them in handfuls to salads. Think of them as leaves packed with plant goodness, rather than just for flavouring – use them generously and go big on taste.

5. Try a new wholegrain or legume in an old-favourite recipe. Not familiar with all the legumes on offer? Turn to my guide on pages 104–105.

Wheel of diversity

This wheel shows just a glimpse of the wide array of options within the Super Six: wholegrains, fruits, veg, nuts and seeds and legumes. We really are spoilt for choice! I'm sure there are some foods on here you already have as a regular part of your diet, and others you've not had for months or perhaps have never tried. Bottom line: it's not exhaustive, it's for inspiration – and one that I bet you can add to!

Not sure what's in season? Head to my website (theguthealthdoctor.com) where there are lists of what's at its best (and also most affordable) by season.

The Diversity Diet toolkit **99**

Wholegrains
- Black pepper
- Amaranth
- Barley
- Buckwheat
- Corn kernels
- Farro
- Freekeh
- Millet
- Oats
- Quinoa
- Rye
- Sorghum
- Spelt
- Teff
- Wheat
- Wheat berries
- Wild rice

Herbs and spices
- Cardamom
- Chilli
- Chives
- Cinnamon
- Coriander
- Cumin
- Fennel
- Ginger
- Mint
- Mustard seeds
- Nutmeg
- Oregano
- Paprika
- Parsley
- Rosemary
- Turmeric

Legumes
- Adzuki beans
- Black beans
- Black-eyed peas
- Borlotti beans
- Broad beans/fava beans
- Butter beans
- Cannellini beans
- Chickpeas
- Edamame/soybeans
- Haricot beans
- Kidney beans
- Lentils
- Lupin beans
- Mung beans
- Pinto beans
- Yellow split peas

Nuts and seeds
- Almonds
- Brazil nuts
- Cashews
- Chia seeds
- Hazelnuts
- Hemp seeds
- Linseed
- Peanuts
- Pecans
- Pine nuts
- Pistachios
- Poppy seeds
- Pumpkin seeds
- Sesame seeds
- Sunflower seeds
- Walnuts
- Watermelon seed

Vegetables
- Artichokes
- Asparagus
- Aubergine
- Beetroot
- Broccoli
- Brussels sprouts
- Carrots
- Cauliflower
- Celery
- Courgette
- Green beans
- Jackfruit
- Leeks
- Mushrooms
- Pak choi
- Peppers
- Spinach leaves
- Sweet potato

Fruit
- Apples
- Apricots
- Bananas
- Blueberries
- Dates
- Figs
- Kiwi fruit
- Limes
- Mango
- Melon
- Oranges
- Peaches
- Pears
- Pineapple
- Plums
- Pomegranate
- Raspberries

Your plant-based shopping list

Increasing your diversity does require you to get a little experimental, inquisitive and imaginative when you hit the shops. I heartily encourage you to shop with the seasons and buy what you fancy when it comes to fresh produce. But when it comes to those store-cupboard staples, the following is a good guide to making sure you're recipe-ready for a plant-based feast.

Flours and powders

- Almond/ground almonds
- Baking powder
- Cocoa powder
- Rye
- Spelt
- Wholewheat

Wholegrains

- Barley
- Buckwheat/soba noodles
- Freekeh
- Jumbo oats
- Mixed wholegrains
- Quinoa
- Sourdough bread
- Wheat berries
- Wholewheat pasta

Fruits and sweeteners

- Coconut flakes
- Cranberries
- Dark chocolate

- Dried apricots
- Dried mango
- Dried figs
- Frozen mixed berries
- Goji berries
- Medjool dates
- Raisins

Nuts and seeds

- Brazil nuts
- Cashews
- Chia seeds
- Ground flaxseed
- Hazelnuts
- Mixed seeds
- Mixed unsalted nuts
- 100 per cent nut butter
- Pecans
- Pine nuts
- Pistachios
- Sesame seeds
- Tahini
- Walnuts

Preserved veg

- ○ Capers
- ○ Frozen mixed veg
- ○ Frozen peas
- ○ Jackfruit
- ○ Jalapeños
- ○ Marinated artichokes
- ○ Nori seaweed
- ○ Olives
- ○ Pickled beetroot
- ○ Roasted peppers
- ○ Sundried tomatoes
- ○ Tinned tomatoes/passata

Herbs and spices

- ○ Chilli flakes or powder
- ○ Cinnamon
- ○ Cumin
- ○ Curry powder
- ○ Garlic
- ○ Ginger
- ○ Mixed herbs
- ○ Nutmeg
- ○ Rosemary
- ○ Smoked paprika
- ○ Thyme
- ○ Turmeric
- ○ Vanilla extract
- ○ Vegetable stock

Condiments

- ○ Coconut milk and cream
- ○ Dijon mustard
- ○ Harissa paste
- ○ Miso paste
- ○ Soy sauce/tamari
- ○ Worcestershire sauce
- ○ Nutritional yeast

Legumes

- ○ Black beans
- ○ Butter beans
- ○ Chickpeas
- ○ Kidney beans
- ○ Mixed beans, in water
- ○ Silken tofu
- ○ Pretty much one of every tin on the shelf!

Oils and vinegars

- ○ Balsamic vinegar
- ○ Cider vinegar
- ○ Extra virgin olive oil
- ○ Sesame oil

Tip

Although it works out cheaper to buy legumes dried, the prep required is a barrier for most. Treat your microbes and go for the tins! Just be sure to pick up the ones in water, not in brine or sauce.

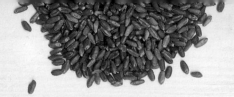

Meet and greet: wholegrains

From the bread you eat and the flour you bake with, to the pasta and rice that accompanies your dinner, it's so easy to get into a rut with wholegrains. If you tend to rely on the same old staples (like wheat, rice and oats), it's time to get acquainted with some of the other deserving options, why they're so great and how you can use them. You may be surprised to find that most of these wholegrains are available in the major supermarkets at no extra cost.

Freekeh
(pronounced FREE-kah)

An ancient type of wheat that's roasted and rubbed to create its flavour.

- **Nutrition need-to-know:** One serving (40g, ¼ cup raw) delivers 4g fibre, 5g protein and 15 per cent of your daily iron needs, plus the plant chemicals lutein and zeaxanthin, which are linked with eye health.

- **Flavour profile and where to use it:** A fluffy and chewy wholegrain with a signature smoky flavour. Ideal for adding texture to soups and salads. Try it in place of couscous.

- **Find it in**: Roasted veg and freekeh salad (page 194)

Buckwheat

Despite its name it's not actually related to wheat. Most commonly found in its wholegrain form (often called a groat), as well as flour and noodles (soba).

- **Nutrition need-to-know:** One serving (40g, ¼ cup raw) delivers 4g fibre, 6g protein and nearly 25 per cent of your daily magnesium needs. A good source of rutin, a polyphenol that packs quite the antioxidant punch and is linked to improved heart health. It's also gluten-free.

- **Flavour profile and where to use it:** With a robust and earthy taste, the wholegrains make a good oat porridge substitute, although soba noodles in a rich soup are my favourite way to eat buckwheat.

- **Find it in:** Stir-fry adventures (pages 216–218)

Spelt

An ancient type of wheat, also known as dinkel wheat.

- **Nutrition need-to-know:** One serving (40g, ¼ cup raw) delivers 5g fibre, 6g protein and over 50 per cent of your daily manganese needs (an essential mineral for the normal workings of your brain and nervous system).

- **What it tastes like and where to use it:** Hearty and slightly nutty, spelt adds more depth of flavour than standard wheat. An easy substitute for standard wheat flour in most baking, both sweet and savoury.

- **Find it in:** Butternut muffins (page 189)

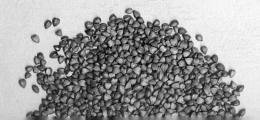
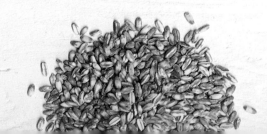

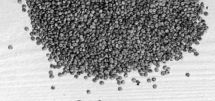

Quinoa
(pronounced KEEN-wah)

Technically a pseudo grain, this is really a seed, but it's prepared and eaten similarly to a wholegrain. There are three main types: white, black and red.

- **Nutrition need-to-know:** One serving (40g, ¼ cup raw) delivers 3g fibre, 6g protein and nearly 20 per cent of your daily folate needs. Quinoa is one of the few plant foods that serves up a complete protein, offering all essential amino acids in a healthy balance. It's also gluten-free.

- **Flavour profile and where to use it:** A mild flavour with a firm texture makes it easy to include at breakfast, lunch or dinner. Ideal for breakfast bowls and saucy dishes. Try it in place of rice.

- **Find it in:** Smoky beet burger (page 213)

Wheat berries

The wholewheat kernel with the food matrix intact, including all three layers: bran (fibre), germ (the nutrient-packed core containing B vitamins and healthy fats) and endosperm (a starchy component with protein). Wholewheat flour also contains each of these elements, they've just been ground up. Whereas white flour just contains the endosperm.

- **Nutrition need-to-know:** One serving (45g, ¼ cup raw) delivers 6g fibre, 6g protein and 15 per cent of your daily zinc needs.

- **Flavour profile and where to use them:** Sweet, creamy yet nutty flavour. The berries hold their shape and keep their chewy bite, which makes them ideal as a barley substitute in soups or for textured rice dishes, as well as being baked into bread to add texture.

- **Find it in:** Flavour of Korea stir fry (page 217)

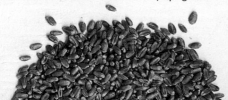

Rye

A close relative of wheat (found in bread, pasta, couscous, etc.) and barley (found in beer, malted products, some multigrain breads and soups), rye is often made into porridge flakes and flour.

- **Nutrition need-to-know:** One serving (40g, ¼ cup raw) delivers 6g fibre and 4g of protein. Rye wholegrains have been shown to have less impact on blood sugar compared to other wholegrains, due to their high levels of viscous arabinoxylan fibre.

- **Flavour profile and where to use it:** Strong, slightly sour yet earthy taste, the flour makes a great substitute for wheat flour in savoury baking such as bread and dense muffins. Best known as the wholegrain behind pumpernickel bread.

- **Find it in:** Seedy cracker duo (page 175)

Red rice

A variety of rice that is naturally coloured red by the polyphenol anthocyanin.

- **Nutrition need-to-know:** One serving (45g, ¼ cup raw) delivers 5g fibre (four times higher than standard white rice) and 4g protein. High in the polyphenol anthocyanin, which is linked with brain health. It's also gluten-free.

- **Flavour profile and where to use it:** Nutty flavour that works well as a substitute in most savoury rice dishes apart from risotto, given its non-glutinous texture.

- **Find it in:** Quinoa rice with hoisin drizzle (page 271)

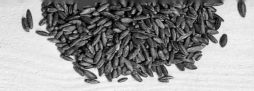

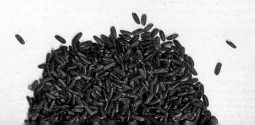

Meet and greet: legumes

Generally speaking, legumes are any plants that grow in pods – including beans and pulses, which are the edible seed within the pods. Along with the early cereal grains, pulses were some of the first crops cultivated, as far back as 11,000 years ago.

All these legumes are widely available and affordable in tins, or even cheaper if you buy dried and soak them. They're also one of the most sustainable sources of protein: good for you, your microbes and the planet, and naturally gluten-free.

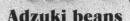

Adzuki beans

Also known as red mung beans, these are popular in Japan in both sweet and savoury dishes.

- **Nutrition need-to-know:** One serving (115g, ½ cup cooked) delivers 8g fibre, 9g protein and nearly 20 per cent of your daily zinc needs. They also pack quite the polyphenol punch, including flavanols linked with skin health.

- **Flavour profile and where to use them:** Subtly sweet and versatile, add these to most dishes, including soups, casseroles and chilli con carne. For something sweet, blend them with your natural sweetener of choice (I love dates) to make the sweet Japanese red paste *Anko*.

- **Find them in:** Leafy taco wraps (page 185)

Butter beans

The name says it all – blending these creamy beans makes the perfect substitute for butter, without all that saturated fat.

- **Nutrition need-to-know:** One serving (95g, ½ cup cooked) delivers 7g fibre, 7g protein and over 20 per cent of your daily manganese needs.

- **Flavour profile and where to use them:** With a soft and buttery flavour, add them to a stew to soak up all the flavour, or try blending them as you would chickpeas to make a winning hummus or mayonnaise replacement.

- **Find them in:** Crispy bacon-shrooms with creamy butter bean hummus (page 144)

Black beans

A staple food in Central and South America that, when eaten with rice, blunts the blood-sugar rise compared to eating just rice.

- **Nutrition need-to-know:** One serving (85g, ½ cup cooked) delivers 8g fibre, 8g protein and 15 per cent of your daily magnesium needs. They're also one of the highest sources of polyphenols within the legume family, owing to the anthocyanins (also found in blueberries) that are largely responsible for their rich black colour.

- **Flavour profile and where to use them:** Floury and mild in flavour, which is why they make a great replacement for flour in moist, gluten-free chocolate brownies and muffins. They also go well in spicy savoury dishes, including burritos.

- **Find them in:** Muffin in a mug (page 138)

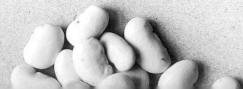

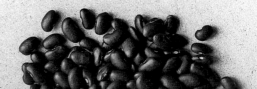

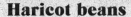

Haricot beans

The infamous baked bean, they are also one of the best sources of fibre in the legume family.

- **Nutrition need-to-know:** One serving (90g, ½ cup cooked) delivers 10g fibre, 8g protein and nearly 20 per cent of your thiamine (vitamin B1) needs.

- **Flavour profile and where to use them:** A little on the bland side, these beans have made their mark thanks to their excellent ability to absorb the flavours of a dish. This makes them ideal to soak up saucy dishes such as tomatoes in baked beans, and stews.

- **Find them in:** Super green pea and 'ham' soup (page 230)

Black-eyed peas

These visually distinct beans resemble eyes, making them a hit with kids. And in the southern United States, eating them on New Year's Day is thought to bring prosperity.

- **Nutrition need-to-know:** One serving (85g, ½ cup cooked) delivers 6g fibre, 7g protein and over 40 per cent of an adult's daily folate needs (not including during pregnancy).

- **Flavour profile and where to use them:** Creamy and earthy, these make a great addition to any dish with rice or couscous. Or fry them in olive oil with garlic, onion and chopped tomatoes as they do in Syria and Lebanon. Yum!

- **Find them in:** Leafy taco wraps (page 185)

Cannellini beans

Also known as white kidney beans thanks to their shape, these come from Italy.

- **Nutrition need-to-know:** One serving (110g, ½ cup cooked) delivers 6g fibre and 7g protein. Like most legumes they're a notable source of iron, but remember to combine with a source of vitamin C such as peppers or tomatoes to help them reach their iron-delivering potential.

- **Flavour profile and where to use them:** With a fluffy texture and slightly nutty flavour, these go perfectly in stir fries and salads. They also make a great switch for short-cut pasta in dishes such as minestrone soup or added to mac and cheese.

- **Find them in:** Creamy beans with 'meaty' jackfruit (page 243)

Pinto beans

You may not recognize these in their dried form, as they lose their specks once cooked, but they are one of the most popular in the United States.

- **Nutrition need-to-know:** One serving (85g, ½ cup cooked) delivers 8g fibre and 8g protein. They are particularly rich in kaempferol, a flavonoid associated with impressive anti-inflammatory benefits, and lowering cholesterol.

- **Flavour profile and where to use them:** Soft with a mild nutty flavour, these versatile beans are often eaten whole, mashed or fried. I recommend them mashed with roasted garlic and onion as a moreish spread.

- **Find them in:** Jacket potato trio (page 196)

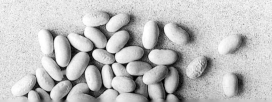

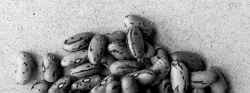

Cooking Tips

- **Boiling, steaming, baking, sautéing, frying . . .** there are many different ways to prepare your plants. I encourage you to mix it up, because they all create different flavours. To maximize nutrient retention, use as little water as possible when poaching and boiling, and don't peel veg until after cooking (better still, don't peel them at all, for more fibre).

- **In a rush?** Steam your root vegetables in the microwave with a splash of water to soften them before baking. This reduces baking time by around 20 minutes.

- **Roast vegetables are so versatile,** so if you're going to the effort of roasting make a double or even triple batch as they last in the fridge for up to five days and make a great addition to most meals (wraps, salads and sandwiches included) and a great snack (try my one-minute sweet potato slider on page 302).

- **Learning to love a new plant?** Be sure to dress it up! See pages 170–173 for some of my favourite dips and pages 216–218 for my favourite stir-fry flavours.

- **Seasoning your plants is quick, tasty** and adds even more plant goodness. Here are some of my favourite flavour combos:

Legumes	Stir fries (see pages 216–218 for my top stir-fry recipes).	Salad dressings	Breads and crackers	Fruits
✓ cayenne	✓ basil	✓ basil	✓ caraway	✓ allspice
✓ chilli	✓ bay leaves	✓ celery seed	✓ cardamom	✓ cardamom
✓ cumin	✓ celery seed	✓ chives	✓ cinnamon	✓ cinnamon
✓ curry	✓ chilli	✓ dill	✓ coriander	✓ cloves
✓ parsley	✓ curry	✓ fennel	✓ cumin	✓ coriander
✓ rosemary	✓ dill	✓ horseradish	✓ dill	✓ ginger
✓ sage	✓ garlic	✓ mint	✓ orange peel	✓ mint
✓ thyme	✓ ginger	✓ mustard	✓ oregano	✓ star anise
	✓ oregano	✓ oregano	✓ rosemary	
	✓ parsley	✓ paprika	✓ saffron	
	✓ rosemary	✓ parsley	✓ star anise	
	✓ smoked paprika	✓ saffron	✓ thyme	

How to read food labels

Another good reason to move towards a more whole plant-based diet is you won't be buying as many packet foods – so there will be fewer labels to decipher (and less plastic waste). When you do, though, it helps if you know what you're looking at.

There are three things worth noting:

1. Don't be misled by the front-of-pack health claims

I don't want to be a downer on your shopping experience or turn you into a sceptic, but those eye-grabbing health claims are often not what they seem. Take the many cereal boxes that shout 'high fibre' and 'immune support' on the front. When you turn them around and dig a little deeper, in more cases than not the fibre comes from a single refined powder such as chicory root fibre (no plant diversity here!) and the added sugars are twice that of the fibre – not to mention the vast collection of food additives.

In terms of immune health, any product with a certain level of micronutrients including vitamin C or B6 can claim that it supports your 'immune health', despite the vast majority of us already getting more than enough of those vitamins from our diets . . . and yes, even those sugar-loaded breakfast cereals with token vitamins added in can make those claims.

2. All the secrets lie in the ingredient list

Forget what the product name is or what it might say on the front; the ingredients list tells you what's really in it. Ingredients are listed from greatest to smallest by weight. So that 'blueberry' cereal bar you bought might have lots of other ingredients higher up the list than actual blueberries (which may feature in a tiny amount, or only as a dried extract or even artificial flavouring, meaning it may never have even seen a blueberry!).

It's worth being an 'added sugar' spy too, because on ingredient lists it often hides in various different disguises: glucose, dextrose, fructose, maltose, sucrose, lactose, syrup (date, maple, corn, brown rice, oat, etc.), coconut blossom nectar, honey, maltodextrin, agave nectar, fruit juice . . . to name just a few. While, yes, a little added sugar is completely fine ('a little' generally means that sugar appears near the end of the ingredient list), don't let them sneak up on you in disguised 'healthy' products.

3. Nutrition information is a comparison game, not about black-and-white rules

Next, you can look to the nutritional information, which is usually displayed in a table, like the one on page 109, and details: fat (including saturates), protein, carbohydrate (including sugars, both naturally occurring and added), salt (often referenced as 'sodium') and energy (measured in both kilojoules and kilocalories). Generally, it'll also list any vitamins and minerals, as well as fibre, if present in significant amounts. Labels will usually give you amounts for these according to serving size, as well as listing the number of servings contained in the overall packet. But beware, this is one of the marketers' favourite tricks – shrinking down the serving size to unrealistically small portions, just to get the pesky calories or sugars down in the table.

As you know by now, I don't typically recommend counting calories or measuring macros like carbs or fat. But I do suggest you get label-savvy, so you can read between the lines and find the products that are best for you. When you're shopping for a product – say, granola – the easiest thing to do is compare products using the 'per 100g' column. That way you avoid the marketing trick of shrinking down the portion size. Most often, the product with the highest fibre and least salt and sugars (especially if the ingredient list suggests it's from added sugars and not whole fruit) makes it into my trolley. In terms of fat and protein, it really depends on the source of these nutrients, e.g. if the fats are coming from whole seeds and nuts (and not refined oils such as palm oil), then in my trolley they go. Again, this is why the ingredient list should be what you pay the most attention to! If you're counting anything, count the number of plants, not calories.

Tip
Aim to buy items that have whole foods listed within the first three ingredients. Added sugars should be low on the list if it's a daily food item.

Sugars: This includes both naturally occurring e.g. from whole fruit and dairy, and added sugars. Avoiding sugar is not necessary, but try to limit larger amounts of added sugars. If sugar content per 100g is more than 15g, check that added sugar is not listed on the ingredients list. Other names for added sugar: glucose, dextrose, fructose, maltose, sucrose, lactose, syrup (date, maple, corn, brown rice), coconut blossom nectar, honey, maltodextrin, agave nectar, fruit juice.

Nutritional information

Servings per package – 5.5

Serving size – 30g (2/3 cup)

	Per serve	Per 100g
Energy	432kj/103kcal	1441kj/344kcal
Protein	2.8g	9.3g
Fat		
Total	0.4g	1.2g
Saturated	0.1g	0.3g
Carbohydrate		
Total	18.9g	62.9g
Sugars	3.5g	11.8g
Fibre	6.4g	21.2g
Sodium	65mg	215mg

Ingredients: Cereals (76%) (wheat, buckwheat, barley), psyllium husk (11%), date syrup, malt extract, honey, rock salt, flavourings, vitamin B6, riboflavin, thiamin

100g Column and serving size: If comparing between similar food products use the per 100g column.

Fibre: Not all labels include fibre. Foods that contain at least 6g of fibre per 100g are considered high in fibre.

Ingredients: Listed from greatest to smallest by weight. Use this to check at least the first three ingredients are whole foods. Remember this is the section you should pay the most attention to.

Sodium (salt): Choose lower sodium options among similar foods. Foods that contain no more than 120mg sodium (0.3g salt) per 100g are considered low in sodium/salt. Other names for high salt ingredients: baking powder, celery salt, garlic salt, meat/yeast extract, monosodium glutamate (MSG), onion salt, rock salt, sea salt, sodium, sodium ascorbate, sodium bicarbonate, sodium nitrate/nitrite, stock cubes, vegetable salt.

Being mindful about eating

Paying a little attention to why and how we're eating goes a long way towards making healthier choices and having better gut health. Have you ever mindlessly eaten a packet of biscuits or a chocolate bar and found yourself, moments later, questioning where it went and second-guessing whether you really did eat the whole thing? Our busy lives have taught us that multitasking is an impressive skill, but this has led to so many of us eating mindlessly. The outcome? We feel less satisfied and are more likely to experience digestive issues. Highly processed foods in particular melt in our mouths (remember how little chewing they require!) so, particularly when distracted, we barely notice we're eating them. And therefore those satiety signals don't have time to register.

Fellow researchers have developed a questionnaire that I often use in clinic to help clients reflect on their current eating habits, drivers and patterns. Head over to theguthealthdoctor.com to complete the questionnaire, and monitor your progress after implementing the ten-step mindful-eating exercise on page 112 for eight weeks.

Revamping your relationship with food

Eating mindfully means being aware, without judgement, of all the physical and emotional sensations of eating. It's a useful tool that can help build a more healthy relationship with foods that may have previously been 'banned' when dieting. If you're concerned that eating more plants will make you feel deprived, or you feel out of control around some foods (yes you, peanut butter), or are struggling with cravings (remember, no food is off limits), I'd recommend making mindful eating part of your toolkit.

Supporting your digestion

For those burdened by gut symptoms such as bloating, mindful eating can be a real game-changer. By tuning into all your senses (sight, smell, feel, sound, taste), your body becomes better prepared for the meal (enzymes are released, blood moves to your stomach, your 'fight or flight' nervous system winds down and your 'rest and digest' nervous system ramps up). In turn, your digestive system is more relaxed and can go about its job more efficiently.

Mindful-eating exercise

I'm certainly not expecting you to do this every time you eat – but I have a feeling once you give it a go and see the difference it makes to your eating experience, as many of my clients have done, you may be inclined to do it more regularly.

The 'eating with all your senses' exercise over the page is a really good one to try with a food you'd normally wolf down. A small bar of chocolate or a cookie, for example, or maybe your favourite meal. The ten-step exercise will walk you through this sensuous way of enjoying it, savouring each mouthful, which is a great way to switch off guilt and gorging, and turn on digestion.

If you're struggling with your relationship with certain foods, at a minimum I'd suggest you do this three times a week using a small portion of those foods. If digestive symptoms are more of your concern, try following the exercise for the first few mouthfuls of your main meal of the day. If you're able to keep doing the exercise regularly you'll start to notice this mindful way of eating naturally becomes your new normal. For more food satisfaction, and less digestive distress, give it a go today!

Getting ready

✓ Sit down at a table.

✓ Clear any clutter, make this just about your food.

✓ Set a place for yourself, even if it's just you, and make it look good – a nice glass, a napkin, the right lighting, some gentle music, it all counts.

✓ Take a few extra moments to present your food well. Put away your phone, tablet, magazine, the crossword – you're just eating.

✓ Take a few moments to breathe deeply into your lower belly, close your eyes, relax.

The exercise:
Ten steps to eating with all your senses

1. Appreciate the look of what's in front of you – the colours, shape and form.

2. Close your eyes to engage more deeply with your other senses.

3. Notice the aroma of what you're about to eat. What does it remind you of? Can you smell different notes? Does your mouth start to water?

4. Take a forkful and your first taste by swiping your tongue over the food. How does it feel?

5. Take your first bite – how does it taste just sitting in your mouth?

6. As you start to chew, be aware of the textures and how they change.

7. Tune into the sounds – is the food bubbling? Fizzing? Is there a loud crunch when you bite into it? Try blocking your ears with your fingers to more deeply engage with the sound of each chew.

8. Focus on the taste. Does it change as the food moves around your mouth and the more you chew?

9. Notice how many times you tend to chew the food before you swallow. Consider its onward journey – can you feel it sliding down? Is there a taste left in your mouth?

10. How does eating this food make you feel? Are you enjoying it?

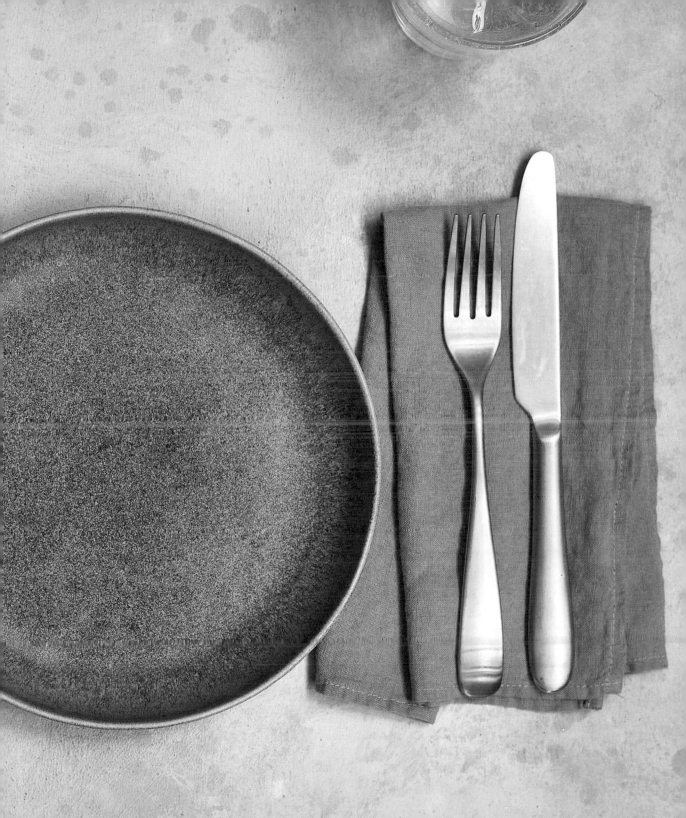

Six tips for adapting to a higher-fibre diet

We touched on how changing your diet in favour of plants might affect those with sensitive guts in chapter 5, but I think all of us would benefit from a little awareness and preparation when it comes to upping our plant portions. Think of it like this: as your diet moves from a little to a lot of fibre, it's naturally going to provide quite the feast for your gut microbes. There may be some excitement, some fizzing and popping – aka that feeling of bloating and gassiness – as your microbes celebrate this new way of eating. But it certainly doesn't have to be that way. If you want to avoid too much gut 'excitement', here are my top tips and tricks to building your tolerance (and your microbes' digestive capacity).

1. Go slow and build up gradually.

Don't transform your diet overnight or binge on plants one day and deprive your microbes the next. Like us, they need 'food' every day to function at their best. If you're worried about how to do this, my menu plan for Sensitive Guts (see page 126) will help guide you.

2. Stay hydrated.

Fibre needs water to 'perform' at its best. So, as you up your fibre, remember to up your water too.

3. Chew your food well.

When it comes to high-fibre whole foods, aim to chew each mouthful around twenty times. This not only helps prep your stomach for the incoming food, but it also kickstarts the digestive process that occurs in your mouth (both physically with your teeth and chemically with the enzymes in your saliva).

4. Keep moving.

Staying active doesn't just support your arm and leg muscles, but your digestive muscles too (remember your digestive tract is wrapped in muscle!).

5. Stretch it out.

Feeling bloated? Some gentle yoga-like stretching at the end of the day can help (when, typically, symptoms are at their peak after a day full of food). Try cat-cow, happy baby and crocodile twist, before resting in child's pose for five deep belly breaths (I demonstrate all of these in *Eat Yourself Healthy*).

6. Worship the heat pack.

For those of you who do experience a little extra gut activity, remember that it is nothing to be worried about. But if it's uncomfortable, applying a heat pack to your stomach can do wonders by drawing extra blood there to support digestion.

De-stressing the gut

Good gut health is not entirely down to diet. There are other factors that can adversely affect your gut health, in particular stress and poor sleep – as those of you with sensitive guts probably know only too well.

A little bit of stress is healthy. Without it, we'd never study for an exam, hit a personal best or achieve many of our goals. But, like all things, there's a fine balance between helpful stress and stress as a hindrance. Whether it's the influx of stress hormones like cortisol playing havoc with our digestive systems, or the angry messages shooting down the communication highway between our brain and gut, chronic stress that niggles at us constantly is a common barrier to good gut health.

A lack of quality sleep is another barrier many of my clients face. Sleep is vital for rest and regeneration, and that goes for your gut too. Indeed, parts of your gut lining shed and regenerate every week or so, and it needs you well rested for this to happen efficiently. Studies have also shown that after just two days of sleep deprivation, your GM is negatively impacted. This is because, like us, our gut microbes have a circadian rhythm (sleep–wake cycle), and if we disturb ours we disturb theirs too.

Thankfully, there are now plenty of research-backed strategies to help us all combat the inevitable periods of stress and poor sleep that modern life throws at us. Check out my seven favourite exercises over the page – they really can make a difference to how you feel.

How to de-stress and sleep better

I know 'reduce stress and sleep better' is hardly useful advice. If it were that easy, I wouldn't be writing this section. So, instead, here's my handy list of evidence-based suggestions that I have seen really work for my clients.

1. Dose up on the cuddle hormone.

Whether it's a hug from someone or one from yourself, the physical sensation of touch has been shown to activate nerves which in turn trigger the increase of oxytocin, the 'cuddle hormone'. This release provides a sense of safety, soothes any feelings of distress and calms that 'fight or flight' sympathetic nervous system. Give it a try, really focusing on how you feel with the initial contact and holding.

2. Self-care is a necessity, not a luxury.

Whether you're tending to your kids' every need, working crazy hours or busy being a good friend . . . you not only deserve but *need* some dedicated 'me-time', or you will absolutely burn out. Whether it's a candle-lit bubble bath or taking yourself on a coffee date (just you), scheduling in at least a couple of thirty-minute self-care sessions in your diary each week is well worth the time investment.

3. Acknowledge and accept your feelings.

Here is one of my favourite quotes, from poet Nayyirah Waheed: 'and I said to my body softly, "I want to be your friend." It took a long breath and replied, "I have been waiting my whole life for this."' Sometimes we run the risk of ignoring or even suppressing our thoughts and feelings. In fact, in clinic I often find gut issues are worse in those whose stress is subconscious. Being able to suppress emotions may be a nifty skill for combating acute stress, but in the long term these emotions often scream out via your gut. How are you feeling right now? Deep down? Acknowledge it's okay to feel that way. Say to yourself out loud, *'I am feeling . . . . . . – and it's okay to feel that way.'*

4. Keep a gratitude diary.

At the end of each day, list three things that happened for which you are grateful. It could be a smile from a stranger, a call from a friend or a nice email from a colleague. As simple as it sounds, reflecting on the good things can 'rewire' how your brain thinks over time, creating more inner peace and calm – no matter your external environment.

5. Do a five-minute body scan.

In a relaxed, seated position, with your eyes closed, imagine a gentle flow of warm liquid light trickling down from above your head through your body, filling up gradually from your pinky toes. Notice the liquid's calming quality filling up your feet, through your ankles, into your lower legs . . . Continue for several minutes to visualize it filling each individual part of your body until it reaches the top of your head. Let it overflow, covering your skin with a warming touch. Slowly open your eyes and reflect on how you feel.

6. Try box breathing.

Breathe in through your nose for four seconds, hold for four, exhale slowly and steadily through your nose for four, hold for four. Repeat for ten cycles. The holding of breath changes the amount of carbon dioxide in the body, which through a sequence of mechanisms activates your 'rest and digest' nervous system, aka your parasympathetic system. The result? A wave of calm moves through your body. Try it!

7. Go forest bathing.

This is just another term for mindfully spending time in nature. Rain, hail or shine, develop curiosity for how your body feels as you walk through nature, as each foot lands on the ground. It's all about being present with those otherwise automatic and unconscious movements. And while 'being with nature' may sound a bit hippie-dippie, a body of research including fourteen studies has shown that forest bathing really does lower stress levels, and even high blood pressure.

Getting started on your journey

It's really up to you how you approach the Diversity Diet. You may want to embrace all the tips in this chapter and dive into my recipes, or perhaps you'd prefer just to dip your toe in, and start by tracking your weekly plant points (see page 29) if you're going for a more gradual approach. Whether you start by focusing on one meal a day – breakfast, lunch or dinner – or just try some of my one-minute snack ideas (see pages 302–303) as an easy win, so long as you're moving in the direction of plant-based diversity, your microbes will absolutely appreciate your efforts.

My approach to food is very practical. The recipes are for you to use every day, and you don't need to be a skilled cook to make any of them (I'm certainly not!). You'll notice a range of features, indicated with icons at the top of the page, including **freezer-suitable** recipes, perfect for batch-cooking ahead of time ready for busy weeks; recipes that can be made **FODMAP-lite** for people with more sensitive guts (see pages 304–308 for detailed switches for each recipe); **fridge raids**, where you use up any fruit and veg that'll soon be on the turn, and **zero-waste** recipes so you can do your bit for saving the planet. There are also a few 'reinvented' recipes where you can use the leftovers of a dinner recipe to create a tasty lunch the next day (pages 205, 207 and 208). My hope is that, after seeing how easy and delicious this way of eating is for yourself, you'll consider cooking for friends and family too – and together discover some of the incredible tastes, textures and experiences you can have by embracing the Diversity Diet.

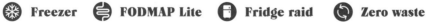 **Freezer**   **FODMAP Lite**   **Fridge raid**   **Zero waste**

I know from experience with clients – and from your messages about *Eat Yourself Healthy* – that lots of you love a little more guidance to help you change your habits. So I've created three different menu plans for different lifestyles – Fuelling Families, Busy People and Sensitive Guts – pick one or try all three. My goal with these menu plans is to act as a blueprint for you to adapt based on the recipes that work best for you, your microbes and your lifestyle. Let's take a closer look . . .

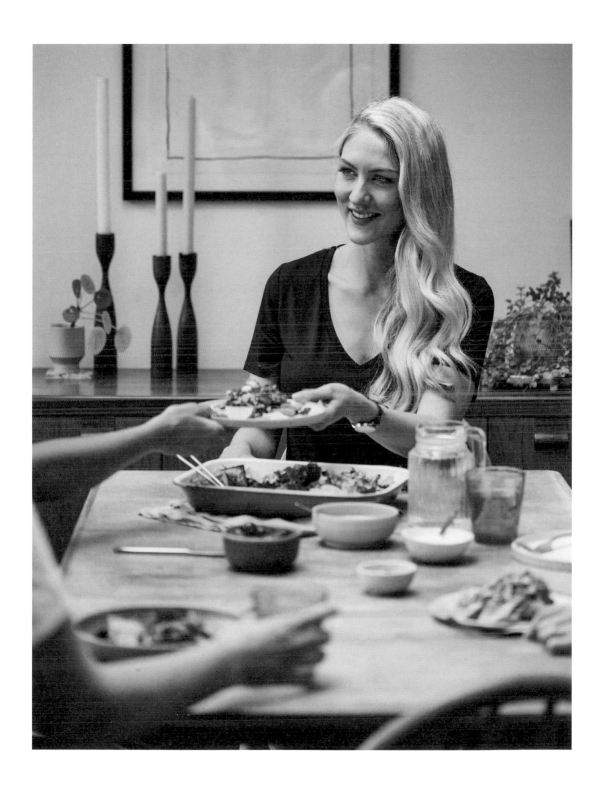

The Diversity Diet menu plans

Plan 1 is for FUELLING FAMILIES
My most versatile, child-friendly meals and fun ideas.

Plan 2 is for BUSY PEOPLE
None of the suggested weekday recipes take longer than twenty minutes to whip up, and many are ready in just five.

Plan 3 is for SENSITIVE GUTS
These all feature FODMAP-lite options (see page 304 for more on this), so you can banish all that plant-based prejudice that often comes with a sensitive gut and start to reap the benefits.

For each plan, I've picked out recipes from the book to give you a whole week's kick-start menu. Each one delivers at least 30 different plant points, along with gut-loving prebiotics, phytochemicals and over 30 grams of fibre per day. In fact, if you follow the plans to a tee, including snacks and desserts, you'll be getting close to 80 plant points across the week and 50 grams of fibre each day! And you'll be happy to know this doesn't mean extra time, complexity or cost on your part. It's all thanks to simple hacks covered on pages 96–97. As you get to know the recipes and what works for you, you can start to build your own menu plan – you can find a printable copy on my website (theguthealthdoctor.com).

I've tried and tested each of these menu plans and found prepping a few recipes on the weekend makes a world of difference for the week ahead, so in each plan I've flagged a few of the recipes worth making in advance. I have designed them to fit around your life instead of your life fitting around them, but feel free to mix and match, and even batch-cook your favourite recipes. I hope they help to steer you as you get going.

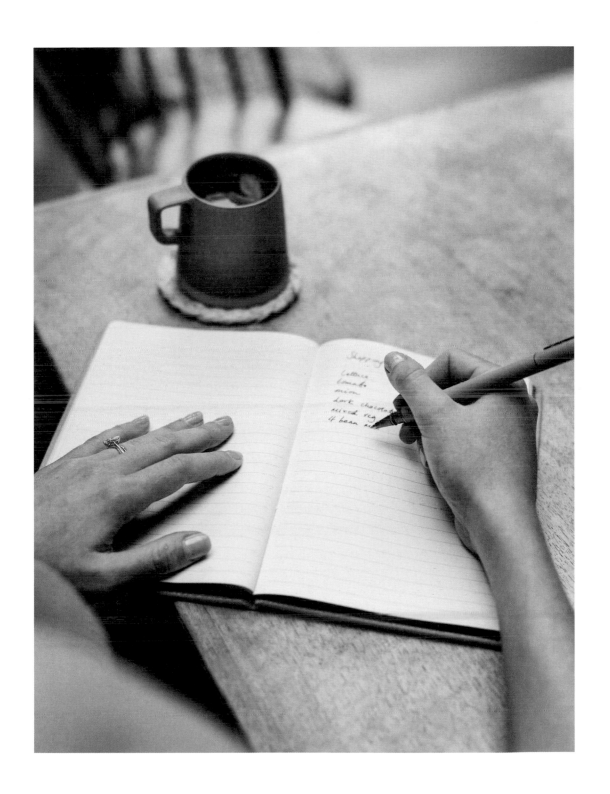

Fuelling families

	Saturday	Sunday	Monday	Tuesday
Breakfast	**Muffin in a mug** (prep DIY plant-packed muesli) (see pages 138, 143)	**Eat-the-rainbow pancake stack** (prep wheaten bread) (see pages 153, 176)	**DIY plant-packed muesli** (made on Saturday) (see page 143)	**Mango and berry fro-yo slice** (made on Sunday) (see page 146)
Lunch	**All-the-greens filo swirl** with **no-added-sugar ketchup** (see pages 180, 173)	**Popcorn chick-less nuggets** with **garlicky aquafaba aioli** **Veg all-dressed-up** (see pages 183, 170, 265)	Sandwich made with **foolproof fermented wheaten bread** (made on Sunday) and toppers of choice (see page 176)	**Sweet jacket potato with nut-free pesto** (see page 197)
Dinner	**Tofu fried wholegrains with crunchy cashews** (see page 202)	**Hearty lasagne** (prep mango and berry fro-yo slice while lasagne is cooking) (see pages 237, 146)	**Stir-fry adventures** (see page 216)	**Spinach and ricotta stuffed pasta shells** (see page 247)

Wednesday	Thursday	Friday
DIY plant-packed muesli (made on Saturday)	**No-bake bites**	**DIY plant-packed muesli** (made on Saturday)
(see page 143)	(see page 142)	(see page 143)
Snack-o-clock veg fritters with **garlicky aquafaba aioli** (made on Sunday)	**Super green pea and 'ham' soup** **Foolproof fermented wheaten bread** (made on Sunday)	*Reinvented* **chicken burger** (using leftover chicken ball mix from Thursday) with **no-added-sugar ketchup** (made on Saturday)
(see pages 179, 170)	(see pages 230, 176)	(see pages 205, 173)
Creamy dairy-free linguine	**Chicken 'n' veg meaty balls** (make a double batch) **Quinoa rice with hoisin drizzle**	**Loaded vegan nachos**
(see page 225)	(see pages 256, 271)	(see page 231)

Snacks & desserts

- **Loaded melon wedges** (page 157)
- **Seedy cracker duo** (page 175)
- **Cream-less ice cream** (prep the day before – page 277)
- **Plant wheels** (page 158)
- **Prebiotic cookie dough drops** (page 163)
- **Choc chip courgette cookies** (page 289)
- **Raspberry red smoothie** (page 295)
- **Prebiotic rocky road** (page 281)
- **Snickers smoothie bowl** (page 293)

One-minute snacks

- **Banana bites** (page 302)
- **Beans 'n' crackers** (use any leftover cashew cheese from Friday) (page 303)
- **Prebiotic 'chocolate' milkshake** (page 302)
- **Apple slider** (page 302)
- **Sweet potato slider** (using leftover sweet potato from Tuesday) (page 302)

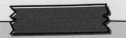

Busy people

	Saturday	Sunday	Monday	Tuesday
Breakfast	Breakfast pitta pizza	Plant-powered baked oat slice or **no-bake bites**	Immunity-nourishing smoothie	Omelette bowl Frothy cashew latte
	(see page 151)	(see pages 148, 142)	(see page 294)	(see pages 139, 300)
Lunch	Thai-inspired fishcakes and crunchy salad	Filo parcels with saucy mushrooms	Leafy taco wraps	Butternut muffins (left over from Sunday)
	(see page 210)	(see page 222)	(see page 185)	(see page 189)
Dinner	Tear-and-share with butter bean relish **Veg all-dressed-up** (optional side)	Butternut muffins	*Reinvented* saucy mushroom pitta pockets (using leftover mushrooms from Sunday)	Stir-fry adventures
	(see pages 248, 265)	(see page 189)	(see page 207)	(see page 216)

Wednesday	Thursday	Friday
Plant-powered baked oat slice or **no-bake bites** (leftover from Sunday)	**Fibre-filled breakfast wrap**	**Muffin in a mug** **Frothy cashew latte**
(see pages 148, 142)	(see page 141)	(see pages 138, 300)
Sweet jacket potato with black beans	**Courgette and hazelnut salad**	**Beetroot, lentil and goat's cheese salad**
(see page 196)	(see page 184)	(see page 193)
Super green pea and 'ham' soup	**Stir-fry adventures**	**Easy noodle broth**
(see page 230)	(see page 216)	(see page 229)

Snacks & desserts

- Trail mix loaf cake with yoghurt and white chocolate glaze (one for the freezer, skip the glaze)
- Stuffed dates
- Cream-less ice cream (no-freeze option)
- Four-ingredient citrus slice

One-minute snacks

- Sweet potato slider (using leftover sweet potato from Wednesday)
- Courgette slider (using leftover pizza base from Saturday as the dip)
- Prebiotic 'chocolate' milkshake
- Fro-yo berries
- Mediterranean stack
- Apple slider
- Banana bites
- Bean dippers
- Avo slider
- Beans 'n' crackers

Don't have a minute? Swap for: fresh fruit; a 150g tub of live yoghurt; a handful of mixed nuts; or hummus with a whole carrot or a stick of celery.

Sensitive guts

	Saturday	Sunday	Monday	Tuesday
Breakfast	Crispy bacon-shrooms with creamy butter bean hummus (see page 144)	Plant-powered baked oat slice Frothy cashew latte (see pages 148, 300)	Fibre-filled breakfast wrap (see page 141)	Omelette bowl (see page 139)
Lunch	Chunky veg and feta frittata (see page 201)	Butternut muffins (see page 189)	Chunky veg and feta frittata (made on Saturday) (see page 201)	Sweet jacket potato with nut-free pesto (see page 197)
Dinner	Orange-glazed roasted salmon and **sticky parsnips** (see pages 226, 264)	All-the-greens filo swirl with **garlicky aquafaba aioli** (see pages 180, 170)	Stir-fry adventures (see page 216)	Chicken 'n' veg **meaty balls** with **quinoa rice with hoisin drizzle** (see pages 256, 271)

Wednesday	Thursday	Friday
Immunity-nourishing smoothie	Plant-powered baked oat slice (made on Sunday)	Muffin in a mug Frothy cashew latte
(see page 294)	(see page 148)	(see pages 138, 300)
Reinvented chicken burger (using leftover chicken balls)	Courgette and hazelnut salad	Butternut muffins (from Sunday)
(see page 205)	(see page 184)	(see page 189)
Thai-inspired fishcakes and crunchy salad	Popcorn chick-less nuggets with garlicky aquafaba aoli (made on Sunday) Veg all-dressed-up	Stir-fry adventures
(see page 210)	(see pages 183, 170, 265)	(see page 216)

Snacks & desserts

- Choc chip courgette cookies
- Ultimate raspberry and white choc muffins
- Trail mix loaf cake with yoghurt and white chocolate glaze
- Seedy cracker duo with a scrape of leftover creamy butter bean hummus (from Saturday) and tomato
- Cream-less ice cream: no-freeze option
- Prebiotic pistachio berry bursts
- Raspberry and lemon ricotta baked cheesecake
- Spinach balls with tahini sauce

One-minute snacks

- Mediterranean stack
- Courgette slider
- Banana bites
- Bean dippers
- Avo slider
- Prebiotic 'chocolate' milkshake

See the FODMAP-lite tweaks and portion guidance, which are detailed for each recipe at the back of the book on pages 304–308.

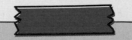

The Diversity Diet toolkit   **127**

FODMAP-lite foods

If you've read my first book, chances are you'll know quite a lot about FODMAPs. But if not, here's a quick recap on the basics, and how they tie into the Sensitive Guts menu plan.

FODMAP is an acronym for a group of carbohydrates, many of which are prebiotic fibres that your gut microbes love to eat. However, for those with more sensitive guts, loading up on too many FODMAPs at once may trigger gut symptoms, such as uncomfortable bloating, extra gas, altered poops and more. The low-FODMAP diet is a medical diet which involves a restriction stage that cuts out all high-FODMAP foods. This has been shown to be effective in providing short-term relief, particularly in people with severe irritable bowel syndrome (IBS).

But there are several risks attached to the strict nature of the diet. So instead, I've developed a much less intensive and lower-risk approach, which I call FODMAP-lite. My approach reduces the FODMAP load – giving sensitive guts more time to adapt without cutting these gut-loving foods out completely.

The recipes with the ⊜ icon can be made FODMAP-lite by making switches and watching the portions outlined for each recipe on pages 304–308. The FODMAP-lite recipes do not restrict lactose, i.e. milk sugar, so if you know lactose is an issue for you then switch to lactose-free yoghurt and milk options. I have also included a list of general FODMAP switches on page 309.

The most common FODMAP-lite switches:

Dates/date paste ➡ maple syrup

Garlic ➡ garlic-infused olive oil

Onion ➡ chives or the green part of spring onions

Wheat, spelt or rye flour and wholegrains ➡ gluten-free flour and wholegrains

---

Soy or oat milk ➡ almond milk

Legumes ➡ tinned legumes, triple-rinsed with water
(stick to 45g, ¼ cup per serving)

If high FODMAP foods are a concern for you, be sure to check out the full FODMAP-lite guide in my first book, *Eat Yourself Healthy*. This includes more information about the reintroduction and personalization stages of the FODMAP-lite approach, which are key to nourishing your gut in the long term.

Plant points planner

Whether you are following the menu plans or not, I have created this planner (example below) for you to keep track of the plant points you eat each week – there is a blank one on my website for you to print off too. The aim is to record the plants you've eaten each day, then tally up your points – turn to page 29 for a reminder of what counts towards your total. Remember that you only record each ingredient once a week, so don't worry if you are just scoring one or two a day by the end of the week – that's normal, especially if you

	Saturday	Sunday	Monday	Tuesday
Date:	25.7.21	26.7.21		
Wholegrains:	Oats, wheat berries	Quinoa		
Fruit:	Dates, red apple, mango	Strawberries, blueberries		
Vegetables:	Beetroot, spring onion, watercress, carrot, celery, purple cabbage	Portobello mushrooms, butternut squash, courgette, sweetcorn		
Nuts & seeds:	Almonds, sunflower and pumpkin seeds	Walnuts, chia seeds		
Legumes:	Chickpeas, butter beans	Soya beans		
Herbs & spices:	Coffee, basil, paprika, EVOO	Garlic, cocoa, cinnamon		
Daily Total:	Plant Points 17	Plant Points 10.75	Plant Points	Plant Points

Week 1

batch cook – it's the weekly total that counts and if you've got above 30 your gut microbes will be thrilled! On each of my recipes I have included how many plant points they provide if you follow them to a tee but make sure to record what you actually ate. For example, if you used mixed seeds rather than just sunflower seeds, remember to count each variety – it all adds up, the more the merrier!

Wednesday	Thursday	Friday
Wholegrains:	Wholegrains:	Wholegrains:
Fruit:	Fruit:	Fruit:
Vegetables:	Vegetables:	Vegetables:
Nuts & seeds:	Nuts & seeds:	Nuts & seeds:
Legumes:	Legumes:	Legumes:
Herbs & spices:	Herbs & spices:	Herbs & spices:
Daily Total:	Daily Total:	Daily Total:
Plant Points	Plant Points	Plant Points

Weekly Total:

Plant Points

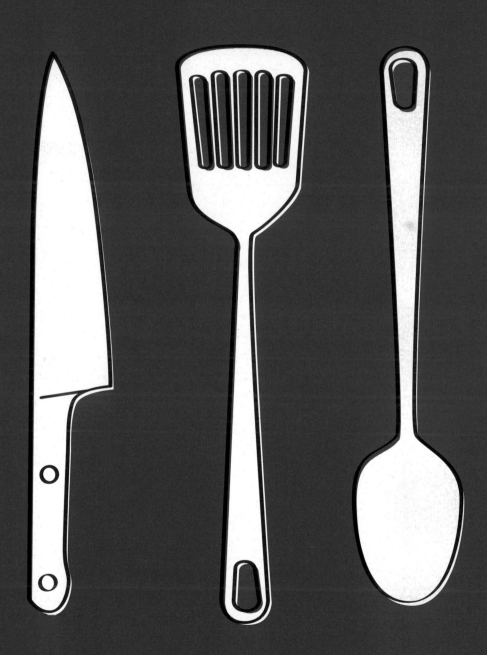

Recipes

A note on ingredients

Peeling

Where I haven't specified peeling your plants, keep the skins on (just rinse well). This will not only save you time, but give you extra fibre too.

Oil

Did you know that it's safe to cook with good-quality extra virgin olive oil (EVOO)? Research has shown it may be even more stable in home cooking (up to 240°C for 20 minutes) than other oils, including sunflower, canola and coconut oil. That's thanks to its high plant-chemical content and its antioxidant powers, which protect the fat from breaking down. Given the wealth of health benefits attributed to EVOO, it's what I recommend using in most of the recipes. (However, feel free to switch it out for your oil/fat of choice, it's your call.)

How do you spot 'good quality' EVOO? Check: 1. The label includes both a best before and a harvest date; 2. It is stored in a dark glass bottle; and 3. It has a certified stamp on it.

Nuts and seeds

Not that into them? Roasting them in the oven or frying pan for two minutes (even if I haven't specified it in the recipe) really does transform the taste and aroma, and gives them that all-important crunch. While it may slightly change the nutritional properties, in the grand scheme of your diet it's rather negligible, especially if the alternative is skipping them altogether.

Sweeteners

Unlike added sugars (see page 107 for a list) whole dates are loaded with both gut-loving prebiotics and other phytochemicals too, such as flavonoids. This is why I tend to use whole Medjool dates as my sweetener of choice in the recipes. Simply mash down one pitted date with 2 tablespoons of hot water until it forms a paste using the back of a spoon. Where the recipe calls for 2 dates, increase the water to 4 tablespoons (¼ cup), and so on. Not fussed? Switch for your sweetener of choice, such as maple syrup or honey (1 date = 1 tablespoon of sweetener = 15 grams).

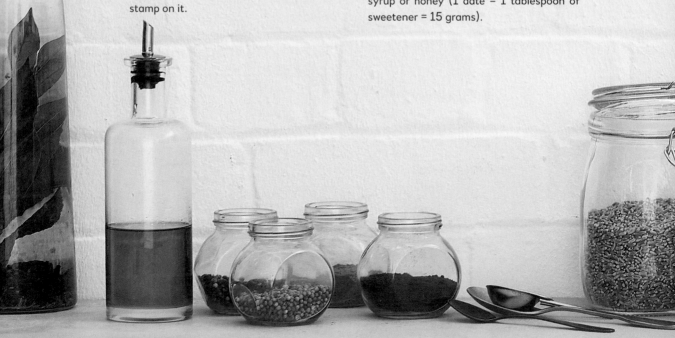

Measurements

Unless specified, ingredient weights are given as prepped weight.

Live yoghurt

Although all yoghurt requires live bacteria to produce it, depending on the processing and storage methods a lot of these bacteria can die before they make it into your shopping trolley. For reassurance that you're getting a decent number of live bacteria, I recommend opting for yoghurts that declare 'live' on the pack (or make your own! For a recipe, see *Eat Yourself Healthy*). I also recommend using yoghurt with no added sugar, sweeteners, thickeners or emulsifiers – just straight up full-fat (whole) milk and live cultures. Why full-fat? Studies have suggested that the fat can help the bacteria survive through our acidic stomachs. And remember, fat is not to be feared. It gives yoghurt an amazing mouth feel, prevents ice crystals from forming when freezing (such as in the mango and berry fro-yo slice recipe on page 146) and can keep you satisfied for longer.

Wholemeal, wholegrain or wholewheat?

Simply speaking, these are all variations of the same thing: wholegrains with all the fibre goodness included. For other flours specified in the recipes such as spelt and rye, ideally opt for wholegrain where you can.

Salt and pepper

Because our taste buds adapt to our use of seasoning, the addition of salt in particular is very personal. I have only listed salt and pepper in the ingredients list where I've specified a set amount. For the other recipes I've just included a note in the methods to 'season to taste'. For me adding a little salt and pepper really does elevate a dish and given much of the salt we eat comes from processed foods, adding a little to your cooking is fine for most (although if you have high blood pressure it's worth reviewing your intake). When it comes to salt, I like to use sea salt, purely based on taste and texture. Despite the myths, it's not any 'healthier'.

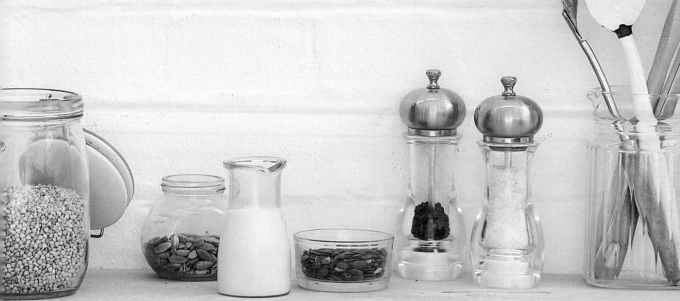

Breakfast

Muffin in a mug

Plant Points
4.25

Serves **2**   Prep **3 mins**   Cook **1.5 mins per muffin**

 FODMAP Lite

For those mornings when a bowl of cereal just won't cut it, looking after your gut health doesn't mean chocolatey goodness is off the breakfast menu. A moreish chocolate muffin with hidden goodies for your gut microbes, including 9g of fibre per portion, no added sugar and ready in minutes . . . what's not to love?

2 large eggs
60g black beans, drained and rinsed
    (approx. ¼ tin)
1 tsp vanilla extract
3 Medjool dates, pitted (approx. 50g)
40g porridge oats
1 ripe banana (approx. 100g)
2 tbsp cocoa powder
1 tsp baking powder

Toppers (optional):
2 squares dark chocolate (approx. 10g)
¼ cup of live yoghurt

Add the eggs to a high-powered blender and blitz for 20 seconds, before adding all of the other ingredients and blitzing for a further 20 seconds until the mix is smooth. Divide into two clean, microwave-safe cups (approx. 250ml capacity). Top with the chocolate (if using), before placing one mug in the centre of the microwave.

Cook on high for 1½–2 minutes, or until it is set on top (it will keep cooking a little as it cools). Repeat with the second mug if cooking for two, or keep it in the fridge for tomorrow.

Allow to cool for a minute before adding a dollop of yoghurt (if using) and tucking in.

Storage You can use your leftover black beans for the loaded vegan nachos recipe on page 231 – or they can be kept in the fridge (best in a container, not the tin) for up to 5 days.

Omelette bowl

Serves **1**   Prep **2 mins**   Cook **3 mins**

 FODMAP Lite

My 'running late for a meeting but craving a savoury breakfast' take on the humble Aussie zucchini (courgette) slice. A hybrid between an omelette and a frittata with almost 7g of fibre – don't shun the microwave for a deliciously healthy and easy way to start your day.

2 large eggs, beaten
¼ tsp onion granules
½ courgette, grated (approx. 90g)
40g frozen peas
25g fetu, crumbled, or cheese of choice
1 slice of seeded bread, torn into small pieces (approx. 40g)
10g pine nuts (optional)

Combine all the ingredients in a microwave-safe dish.

Microwave on high for 2 minutes. Stir the mix, and heat for a further minute. If the eggs are still runny, continue to microwave in 20-second bursts until just set; it will keep cooking a little as it cools. Don't worry if it puffs up a lot in the microwave, it will sink back down.

Allow to cool for a minute before tucking in.

Switch Already had courgette and peas this week? Swap them for 130g of frozen mixed veg of choice.

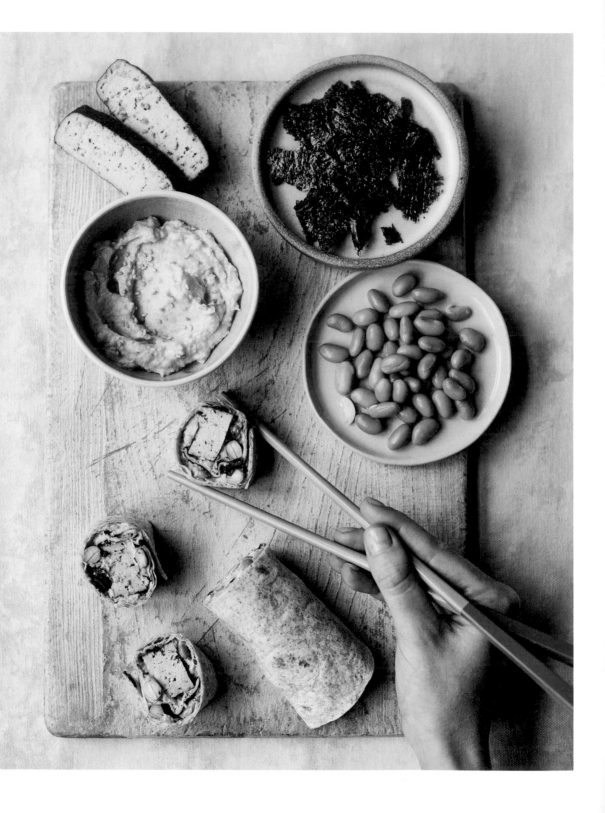

Fibre-filled breakfast wrap

Makes **1 wrap**   Prep **5 mins**

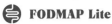 FODMAP Lite

Inspired by Japanese norimaki sushi, where rice and fillings are placed in seaweed (nori) and rolled (maki), this recipe offers an impressive 12g of fibre per portion – that's around four times your traditional nori roll. Spread, sprinkle, wrap and go!

100g smoked tofu

½ avocado (approx. 80g flesh)

1 tsp sesame seeds

2 tsp live yoghurt or vegan aioli (see garlicky aquafaba aioli recipe on page 170)

1 tsp sesame oil

¼ tsp wasabi (optional)

40g edamame beans, fresh, tinned or frozen

½ sheet nori seaweed, crumbled (optional)

1 wholemeal wrap, or wrap of choice

Cut the tofu into two 2cm-wide rectangular logs and set aside.

Mash together the avocado, sesame seeds, yoghurt, sesame oil, and wasabi (if using). Taste, and season to preference, before spreading all over the wrap. Sprinkle the edamame and crumbled nori (if using) on top.

Lay the tofu along one side-edge of the wrap and then roll to encase it.

Cut into five pieces, about 3cm wide, and enjoy.

Tip   No smoked tofu? Fry your own in sesame oil for 2–3 minutes on each side. Prefer a warm breakfast? Heat the tofu strips and edamame beans in the microwave for 1 minute before layering on.

Switch   Prefer a lighter breakfast? Switch out the wholemeal wrap for a sheet of nori seaweed.

No-bake bites

Plant Points
12.5

Makes **12 balls or 4 breakfast bars**   Prep **15 mins**

 FODMAP Lite   **Freezer**

On-the-go breakfast bites with a hit of fruit, veg, wholegrain, nuts and seeds. These are ideal to make ahead of time, freeze, and then grab as you're running out of the door in the morning. Unlike dense and overly sweet energy balls, this lighter version – delivering over a third of your daily fibre needs – will keep you and your microbes satisfied for longer.

75g dried apricots
2 tbsp almond butter, or nut butter
   of choice
30g desiccated coconut
1 tbsp mixed seeds
50g porridge oats
1 tsp ground cinnamon
½ tsp ground ginger (optional)
½ small apple, grated (approx. 50g)
1 carrot, grated (approx. 70g)

Toppers (optional):
30g mixed nuts, crushed
30g desiccated coconut

Place all the ingredients, except for the apple and carrots, in a food processor (apricots, almond butter, coconut (30g), seeds, oats and spices) and blitz for 1 minute or until well combined. Add in the apple and carrot and pulse a couple of times, to roughly combine.

Divide the mix into 12 portions (approx. 25g each) – or if making the breakfast bars, 4 portions. Use your hands to shape each one into a ball/breakfast bar, and then (if using the toppers) roll the ball/bar in mixed nuts, desiccated coconut or both.

Storage These can be kept in the fridge for up to 5 days, or in the freezer for up to 3 months.

DIY plant-packed muesli

Plant Points **18.5**

Makes **20 x 50g portions**   Prep **10 mins**   Bake **25–35 mins, depending on toppers**

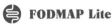 **FODMAP Lite**

An essential for every store cupboard, this is best made at the start of the week so you can just pour and dive in on those busy weekdays. It can also easily be turned into granola for mornings when you fancy a little extra crunch.

Base:
100g raw quinoa
100g coconut flakes, toasted
100g mixed seeds
100g mixed nuts, roughly
    chopped
250g whole oats
100g flakes of choice
    (quinoa, rice, corn, rye)
100g dried mango, chopped
100g dried apple, chopped
100g dried goji berries

Toppers (optional).
2 parsnips or carrots, washed
    and coarsely grated
    (approx. 300g)
2 tsp ground cinnamon
1 tsp ground ginger
1 x 400g tin of chickpeas, or
    legume of choice, drained
    and rinsed

Serving suggestions:
Berries
Live thick yoghurt
Milk of choice

Granola:
4 Medjool dates, made into
    a paste (see page 134), or
    4 tbsp sweetener
3 tbsp extra virgin olive oil

Storage Keep in a cool, dark place, in an airtight container, for 2 weeks.

If including the plant toppers, preheat the oven to *180°C/160°C fan/gas mark 4* and line two large baking trays with paper.

Lay out the parsnip or carrot on some kitchen roll and pat dry, before combining with the cinnamon and ginger and spreading out across one of the baking trays. Repeat the drying process with the chickpeas before spreading across the second tray.

Place both trays in the oven for 20 minutes, before shuffling and baking for a further 15 minutes or until completely dried out. Remove from the oven and allow to cool (ideally left overnight). Be sure to dry the parsnips/carrots and chickpeas out completely, otherwise they will turn the flakes stale.

For the quinoa, heat a large saucepan over a medium-high heat. Once hot, add the grains in a single layer. Shake over the heat until you see them popping, but be careful not to let them burn (don't leave them). They will usually pop within a few minutes. They won't be dramatic like popcorn, but will become tender and deliciously nutty. Allow to cool completely.

Mix together all the remaining muesli base ingredients in a large mixing bowl, adding the now completely cooled dried veg, chickpeas and the puffed quinoa.

Serve with berries, live yoghurt or milk of choice, and if not using the veg toppers, a little shake of cinnamon and ginger to taste.

To turn this into granola

Combine the date paste and olive oil in a bowl before adding in half the muesli mix. Using clean hands, toss to coat the muesli before spreading it across two baking trays lined with non-stick baking paper.

Place in the oven for 10 minutes, toss, then bake for a further 10 minutes or until crisp and golden. Allow to cool completely before transferring to an airtight container.

Crispy bacon-shrooms with creamy butter bean hummus

Serves **2**   Prep **20 mins**   Cook **20 mins**

 FODMAP Lite

I created this recipe to demonstrate to bacon-lovers that plants can be equally as flavoursome. The smoky, crunchy mushroom pieces paired with the creamy butter bean hummus really hit the spot – just ask my meat-loving husband. Offering 50 per cent of your daily fibre needs per portion, you'll be well on your way to smashing your fibre goals.

1½ tsp Worcestershire sauce
1 tbsp red miso
1½ tsp soy sauce
1 Medjool date, made into a paste (see page 134), or 1 tbsp sweetener
2 portobello mushrooms, roughly diced (approx. 130g)

Butter bean hummus (makes 230g, 4 portions):
1 x 400g tin of butter beans, drained and rinsed
1 garlic clove
3 tbsp tahini
juice of ½ lemon (approx. 20ml), to taste
50ml extra virgin olive oil, plus more to taste
1 tbsp nutritional yeast (approx. 5g) (optional)

To serve:
16 cherry tomatoes, ideally on the vine
50g kale
1 tsp extra virgin olive oil
4 slices seedy sourdough, or bread of choice

Preheat the oven to *220°C/200°C fan/gas mark 7*, and line two baking trays with non-stick baking paper.

First, make the vegan bacon-shrooms. In a bowl, mix together the Worcestershire sauce, red miso, soy sauce and date paste. Add the mushrooms and coat them well with the marinade. Spread the mushrooms out on one of the baking trays and drizzle with any leftover marinade, then place in the hot oven for 20 minutes, giving them a stir after 10 minutes.

While the mushrooms are in the oven, place the butter beans, garlic and tahini in a food processor, with half the lemon juice and half the olive oil. Blitz to a smooth paste, and slowly add in the rest of the oil until you have the consistency you prefer. Stir in the nutritional yeast before tasting and flavouring with more lemon juice and seasoning. Put to one side.

Place the tomatoes and kale on the other lined tray, drizzle with olive oil and season. When the mushrooms are nearly cooked, place the kale and tomatoes in the oven and bake for 5 minutes, until the kale is just starting to crisp and the tomatoes are softening a little. The kale cooks very quickly, so keep an eye on it.

Toast the sourdough, spread with some of the butter bean hummus, and top with the vegan bacon-shrooms, kale and tomatoes.

Storage There will be leftover hummus, but this keeps in the fridge for approx. 5 days and is great as a dip or in sandwiches.

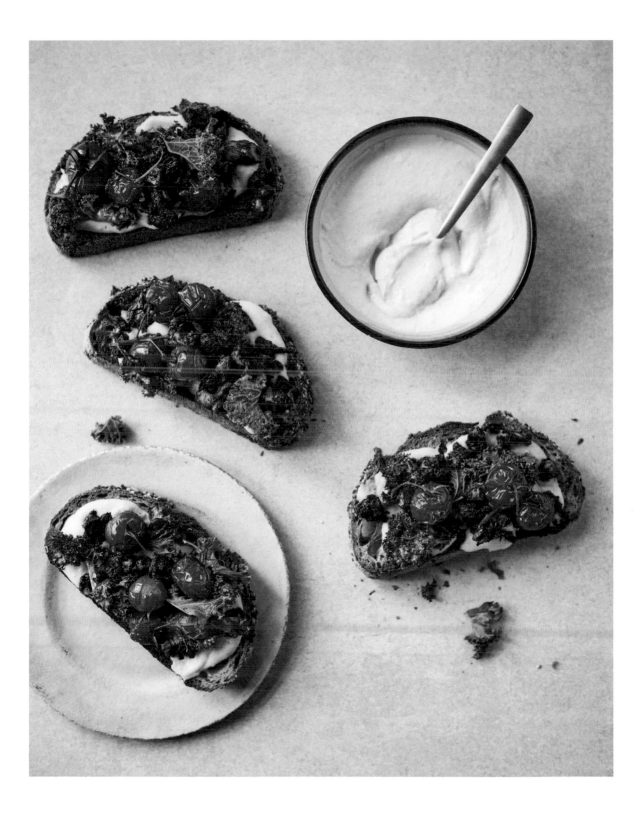

Mango and berry fro-yo slice

Plant Points
5.25

Serves **6**   Prep **10 mins, plus freezing**

 FODMAP Lite   **Freezer**   **Zero waste**

A gut-loving twist on your standard granola and yoghurt breakfast, this recipe can be made as a slice or an ice lolly. Although perfect for a refreshing breakfast, it will double up as your go-to summertime snack.

300g frozen mixed berries, or berries
 of choice
800g live thick yoghurt
400g frozen mango
3 large very ripe bananas, frozen
 (approx. 360g)
1 tsp turmeric

Topper:
185g no-added-sugar granola (see
 page 143 for recipe)

Line a 30cm x 20cm x 5cm tray or dish with non-stick baking paper, or prepare your lolly moulds.

Place the berries in the bottom of the tray (or moulds) and squash a little with a fork. Then place the yoghurt, mango, banana and turmeric in a high-powered blender and blitz for 30 seconds or until smooth.

Pour the mixture into the tray over the berries, and level it out with a spoon or spatula. Sprinkle the granola on top, gently pressing it down into the mix to make sure it sticks when it freezes.

Place in the freezer as soon as possible to prevent the semi-frozen mix from melting (this will help prevent ice crystals forming) and leave – ideally overnight – until it is fully set.

When ready to serve, remove the tray from the freezer 10 minutes beforehand, to allow it to soften a little. Use the paper to lift out the slab and cut into portions before tucking in.

Storage Freeze the individual portions in an airtight container between layers of non-stick baking paper for up to 2 weeks.

Tip Why full-fat yoghurt? The fat is not only thought to protect the microbes as they travel through your acidic stomach, but also makes for a creamier base.

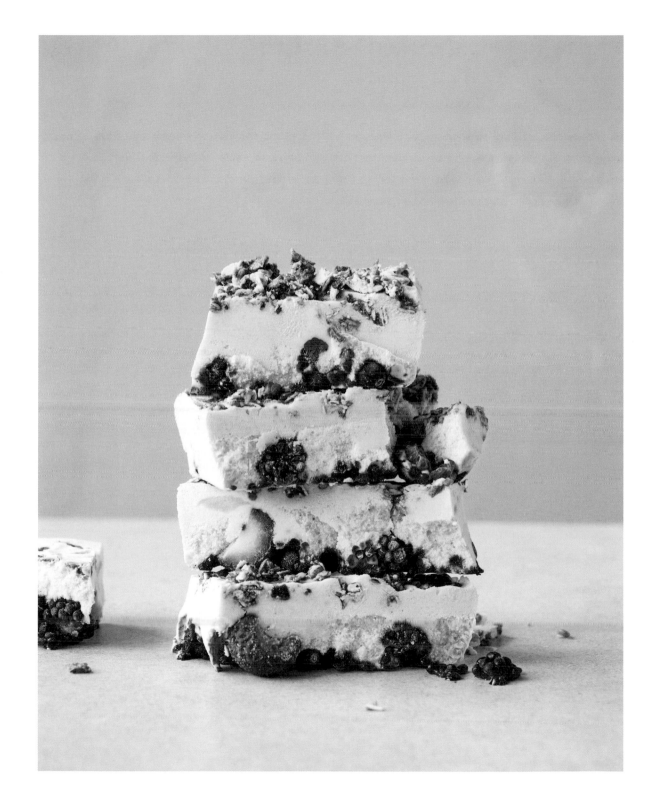

Plant-powered baked oat slice

Plant Points
11.5

Makes **8–10 slices**   Prep **15 mins**   Cook **50 mins**

 FODMAP Lite   ▯ **Fridge raid**   ✳ **Freezer**

My favourite on-the-go slice, loaded with prebiotics, plant points and double the fibre of most breakfast slices. I make a batch at the start of the week and wrap as individual portions, so they're ready to grab as I'm heading out of the door. Hearty, moist and oh-so-satisfying alongside my morning cashew latte (page 300).

1 x 400g tin of cannellini beans, drained and rinsed
2 Medjool dates, made into a paste (see page 134), or 2 tbsp sweetener
3 very ripe bananas (approx. 300g)
300ml soy milk, or milk of choice
200g whole oats
2 tbsp ground flaxseed
1 tbsp ground cinnamon
2 tsp vanilla extract
2 carrots, grated (approx. 140g)
50g raisins, or dried fruit of choice
30g dark chocolate chips
100g frozen raspberries, or berry of choice

Toppers:
50g frozen raspberries, or berry of choice
1 tbsp mixed seeds (optional)

Preheat the oven to *200°C/180°C fan/gas mark 6*.

In a food processor, combine the beans, date paste, bananas and half the milk until roughly blended (approx. 30–45 seconds). Transfer to a large mixing bowl and add in all the additional base ingredients, stir well.

Lightly grease a baking dish (approx. 30cm x 25cm x 3cm) and pour in the mix. Sprinkle over the toppers and gently press down into the mix.

Bake for 45–50 minutes until golden brown and the berries have started to burst. Cover with foil towards the end if over-browning.

Allow to fully cool before serving or storing.

Switch Already had carrots this week? Replace with 140g of courgette.

Storage Can be kept in the fridge for up to 4 days, or in the freezer for up to 3 months. Cut into individual portions before freezing.

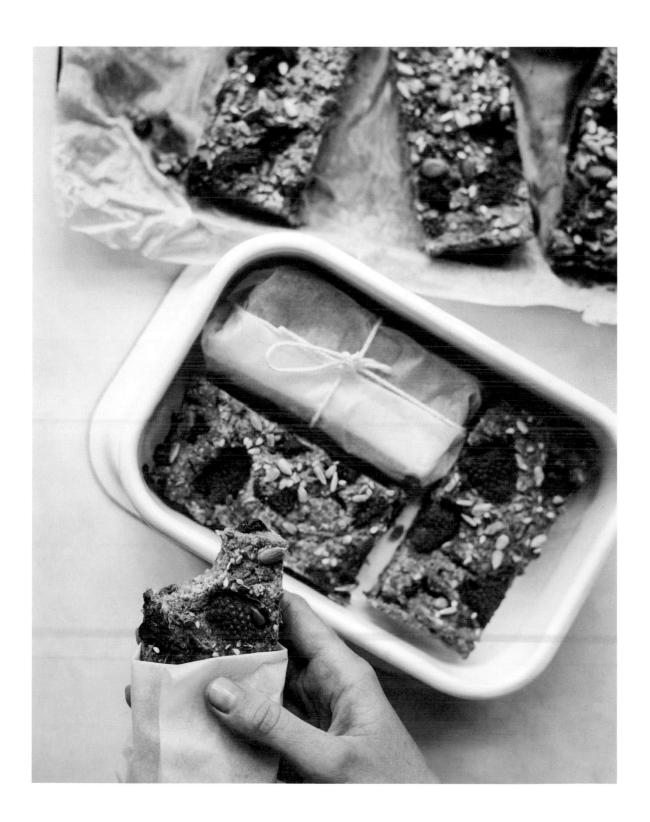

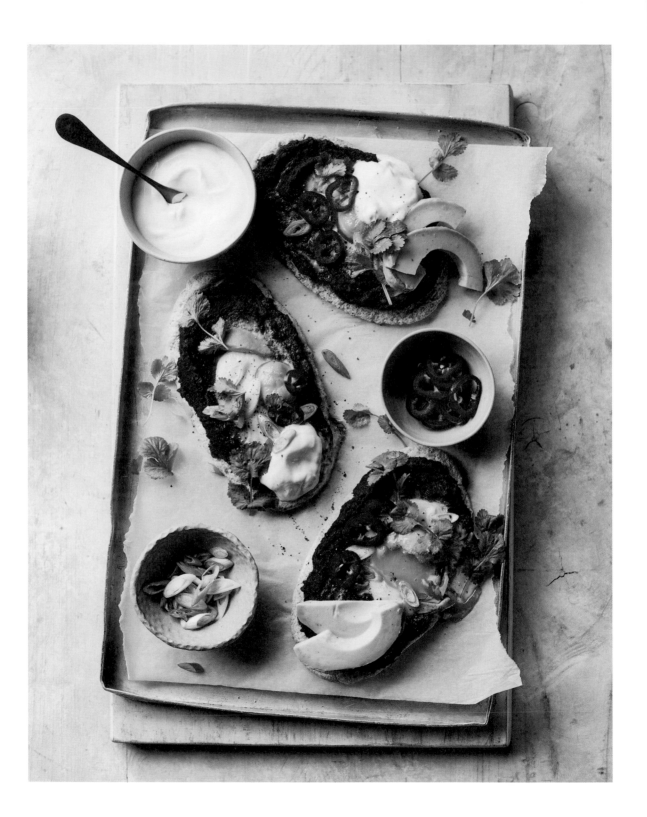

Breakfast pitta pizza

Serves **4**   Prep **10 mins**   Cook **8 mins**

 FODMAP Lite   **Fridge raid**

Who doesn't love the idea of pizza for breakfast? With a rich and tomatoey prebiotic base, this high-fibre pizza (boasting 12g per pizza!) goes perfectly with a gooey egg and any leftover greens or veg from the night before.

4 oval wholemeal pittas

Tomato base:
½ x 400g tin of kidney beans
10 sundried tomato halves, preserved in oil (approx. 85g)
60g pickled beetroot with 3 tbsp brine
1 spring onion, roughly chopped

Toppers (optional):
4 large eggs
1 red chilli, sliced
1 spring onion, finely chopped
3 tbsp live thick yoghurt
1 avocado, sliced (approx. 160g prepped)
10g fresh coriander

Other serving suggestions:
Leftover cooked veg
Flaked salmon
Mackerel
Parmesan shavings
Pine nuts
Capers
Peppers
Salad leaves
Olives

Preheat the oven to *240°C/220°C fan/gas mark 9.*

Lay the pittas on a lined baking tray.

In a food processor, blitz together all the ingredients for the tomato base until you have a smooth paste. Use a splash of water to thin it out if needed.

Spread a quarter of the tomato mixture over each of the pittas, with a thicker layer around the edge to prevent the egg sliding off the pitta. Crack an egg (if using) into the centre of each pitta.

Place the tray in the hot oven for 8–10 minutes or until the eggs are cooked to your liking. Remove from the oven and add the optional toppers of choice (I've gone for chilli, spring onion, a dollop of live yoghurt, avocado and fresh coriander). Season to taste.

Storage Any leftover tomato base can be used as a dip, spread on sandwiches, or sauce on pasta, etc. Store in an airtight container in the fridge for up to 5 days.

Switch I tend to add leftover cooked veg, but if you've only got raw veg, add a drizzle of olive oil to a large frying pan over a medium-high heat and cook the veg for 5 minutes until they start to soften. This helps to remove some of the moisture, saving you from a wet pizza. Add the softened veg, and other toppers that you prefer warm, to your pitta before placing it in the oven.

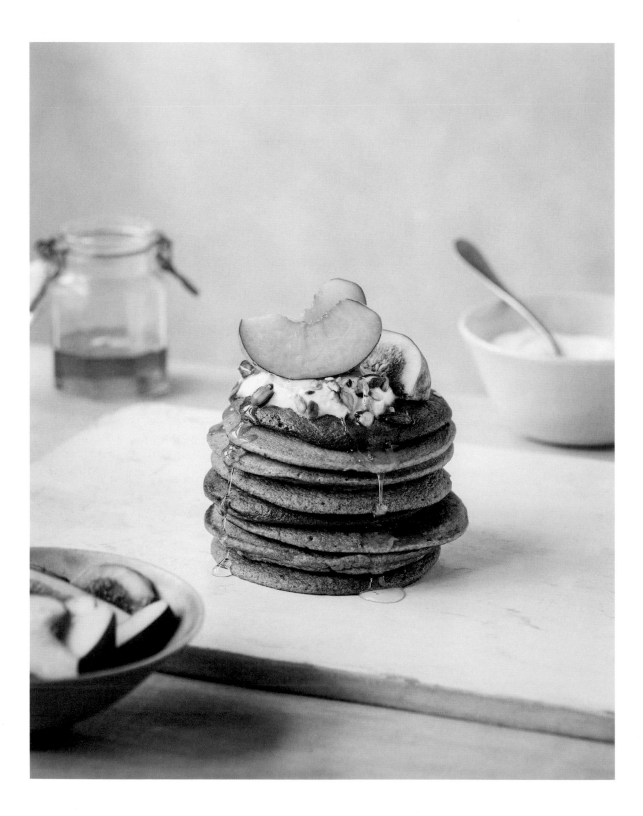

Eat-the-rainbow pancake stack

Plant Points
8.25

Makes **8 small pancakes**   Prep **5 mins**   Cook **15 mins**

FODMAP Lite   ❄ **Freezer**

Nature features so many amazing colours, and this family-favourite breakfast celebrates just that. Alongside the array of gut-loving phytochemicals with their brilliant tones, these rainbow pancakes have just four simple base ingredients and not a food dye in sight. Ease, taste and gut-love flipped into one!

Base:
2 large eggs
2 ripe bananas (approx. 200g)
50g porridge oats
extra virgin olive oil, for frying

Colourings (choose 1 per base):
a. *Pretty Pink (betalain)*
   25g raw beetroot
b. *Mellow Yellow (curcumin)*
   1 tsp turmeric
c. *Proud Purple (anthocyanin)*
   40g red cabbage
d. *Go Green (chlorophyll)*
   30g baby spinach leaves

Toppers (optional):
Live yoghurt, sweetened with honey
Fresh figs
Grilled banana
Berries, blitzed
Toasted mixed seeds

Place the eggs, bananas and porridge oats, along with one of your plant colourings, in a high-powered blender. Blitz for 1–2 minutes until smooth and a little foamy on top.

If you are making additional batches using different colourings (as I've done in the image on page 152), pour the first batch into a jug and set aside. Rinse the blender and repeat the step above.

Heat a large frying pan (or two) with olive oil over a low heat, before spooning in approx. 45ml (or 3 tbsp) of the batter per pancake.

Cook over a low heat for 2–3 minutes, until you see the top of the pancake start to bubble and dry round the edges. This signals it is ready to flip it and cook the other side for another couple of minutes. Don't be tempted to increase the heat level, otherwise you'll lose the vibrant colours.

Repeat until you have used up all the batter. Enjoy with your toppers of choice.

Storage Best eaten straight away – but can be kept in the fridge for 3 days, or frozen for up to 1 month layered between pieces of non-stick baking paper in an airtight container.

Sweet treats

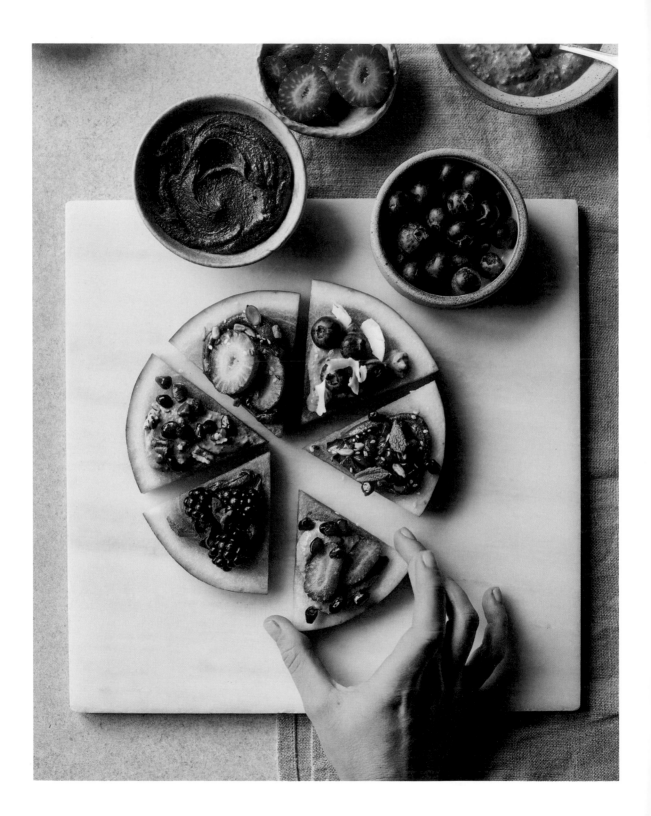

Loaded melon wedges

Plant Points
9.5

Serves **4** Prep **10 mins** Cook **10 mins (if making hazelnut spread)**

FODMAP Lite   **Fridge raid**

Turn snack time into a fun family activity that brings everyone together to create their own watermelon masterpiece. Get creative with the toppers to celebrate the bursting colours of plants and the indulgent flavours of cocoa and hazelnuts.

2 large slices of watermelon or melon of choice, approx. 2cm thick

a. Berry whip spread:
100g blackberries (or cherries, deseeded, approx. 16)
100g ricotta
a touch of honey, to taste (optional)

b. Choc hazel spread:
200g hazelnuts
100g dark chocolate (min. 70%)
1 tsp vanilla extract

Toppers (optional):
Coconut flakes
Blueberries
Strawberries
Pecans
Mixed seeds
Fresh herb leaves (like mint)
Pomegranate seeds

Cut each slice of watermelon into 8 triangles (or 6 if you have a smaller melon).

To make the berry whip spread, use a hand blender to blitz together the berries, ricotta and honey (if using). Set aside.

To make the choc hazel spread, preheat the oven to *180°C/160°C fan/ gas mark 4*. Spread the hazelnuts out on a tray and roast for 5 minutes until lightly golden. While the nuts are in the oven, break the chocolate into pieces and place in a heatproof mixing bowl. Melt by either placing over a pan of simmering water or heating in a microwave in 30 second bursts.

Place the hazelnuts in a high-powered food processor. Blend for 10–15 minutes until a smooth nut butter has formed. Scrape in the melted chocolate and add the vanilla extract. Blitz for another few seconds until well combined and glossy.

Top the wedges of melon with either spread, along with your choice of toppers. I've listed some of my favourites here.

Tip Keep your watermelon in the fridge before serving, for an extra-refreshing slice.

Storage The berry whip spread keeps in the fridge for up to 24 hours and the choc hazel for up to 2 weeks in an airtight jar.

Plant wheels

Makes **18 wheels**   Prep **15 mins plus chilling time**

 Freezer

This glossy fruit log is packed full of plant diversity – with fruits, nuts and seeds all rolled up into one moreish package. It's one of my favourite recipes to showcase that plant-based doesn't mean boring. It's also a great way to diversify high-fibre snacks for kids, and chances are you might already have the ingredients in your cupboard.

120g soft dried figs
120g soft dried apricots
25g walnuts, roughly chopped
40g pistachios, roughly chopped
15g mixed seeds
30g ground almonds
15g dried cranberries
15g coconut flakes

For rolling (optional):
10g desiccated coconut

Place the figs and apricots in a food processor and blitz into a paste. It will take 1–2 minutes and you may need to scrape the sides down. Once ready, it usually makes a thick ball.

Place the walnuts, pistachios and mixed seeds in a dry frying pan over a medium heat. Toast for 2–3 minutes, stirring regularly to prevent burning.

Transfer the fig and apricot paste to a mixing bowl along with the ground almonds, cranberries and coconut flakes and, once cooled, the toasted nuts and seeds. Use a wooden spoon to start the mixing. You will need to press and turn repeatedly to help coax it together, and then finish with your hands.

On a clean work surface, lay out a long piece of cling film. Shape the mix into a long sausage approx. 5cm in diameter. Sprinkle the desiccated coconut (if using) on to the cling film and roll the sausage until coated.

Wrap the sausage tightly in the cling film, twisting the ends to make it airtight, and pop it in the freezer to harden for at least 4 hours. To serve, unwrap it (while still frozen) and use a sharp knife to cut it into 18 mini-wheels.

I love eating the wheels straight from the freezer, but store in the fridge if you prefer a softer texture. Enjoy!

Storage   Store in the fridge in an airtight container for up to 2 weeks or freezer for up to 2 months.

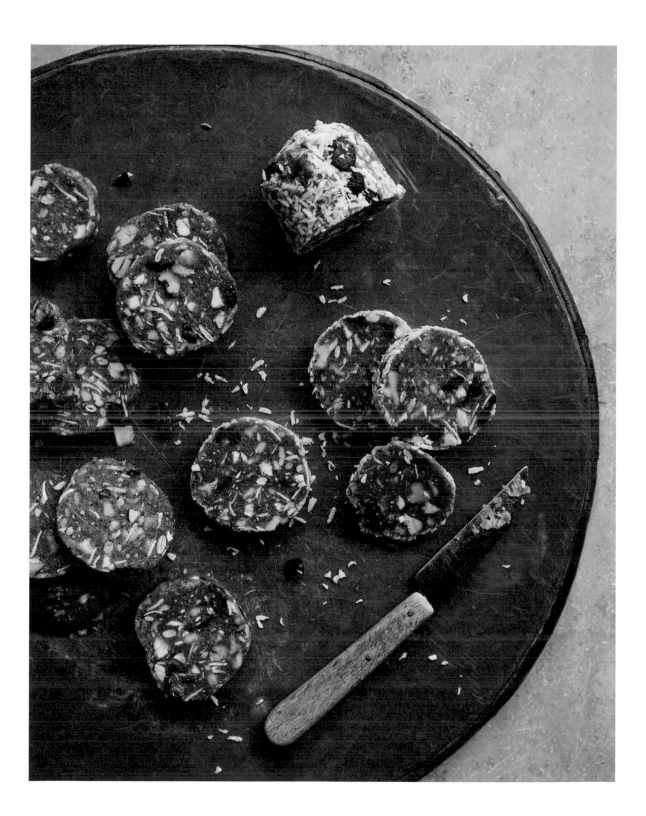

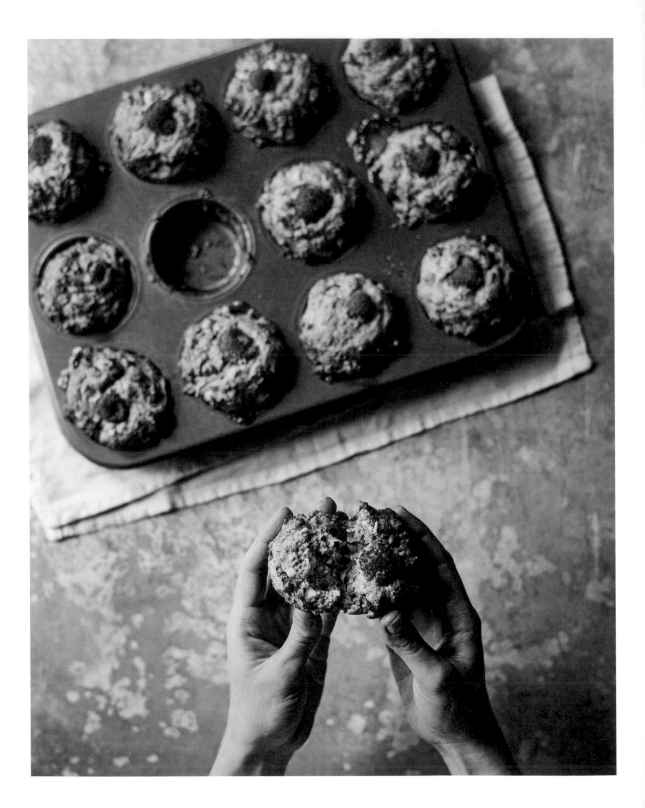

Ultimate raspberry and white choc muffins

Makes **12 muffins**   Prep **15 mins**   Cook **25 mins**

 FODMAP Lite   ❄ **Freezer**

Inspired by the muffins I used to get from my local bakery, these muffins combine my two favourite things: white chocolate and plants! The raspberries are a top source of gut-loving polyphenols too. What's more satisfying than a sweet, moist muffin, and knowing that you're 5.5 plant points closer to your 30 for the week?

3 large eggs, beaten

150g live thick yoghurt

2 tsp vanilla extract

60ml extra virgin olive oil

3 Medjool dates, pitted and roughly chopped (approx. 50g), or 3 tbsp sweetener of choice

1 very ripe banana (approx. 100g)

275g spelt flour, or wholemeal flour

2 tsp baking powder

1 tbsp poppy seeds

100g white chocolate chips

150g grated carrot (approx. 2 carrots)

100g frozen raspberries

To decorate:

12 raspberries, frozen or fresh (approx. 40g)

Preheat the oven to *190°C/170°C fan/gas mark 5*. Grease a 12-hole muffin tin and add a disc of non-stick baking paper to the bottom of each to prevent sticking.

Blitz the eggs in a food processor for 30 seconds until a little foamy. Add in the yoghurt, vanilla extract, olive oil, dates and banana, and blitz for 30 seconds or until smooth.

In a large bowl, mix together the flour, baking powder, poppy seeds and chocolate chips. Then pour in the wet mix from the food processor, followed by the carrot and raspberries. Combine into a thick batter.

Fill each muffin hole evenly with batter (approx. ¼ cup). Push one raspberry into the top of each muffin, before placing the tin in the oven.

Bake the muffins for approx. 25–30 minutes, or until a skewer comes out clean (minus any melted white chocolate), then place the muffins on a wire rack to cool before tucking in!

Storage   These can be kept in an airtight container for 3 days or frozen for up to 3 months.

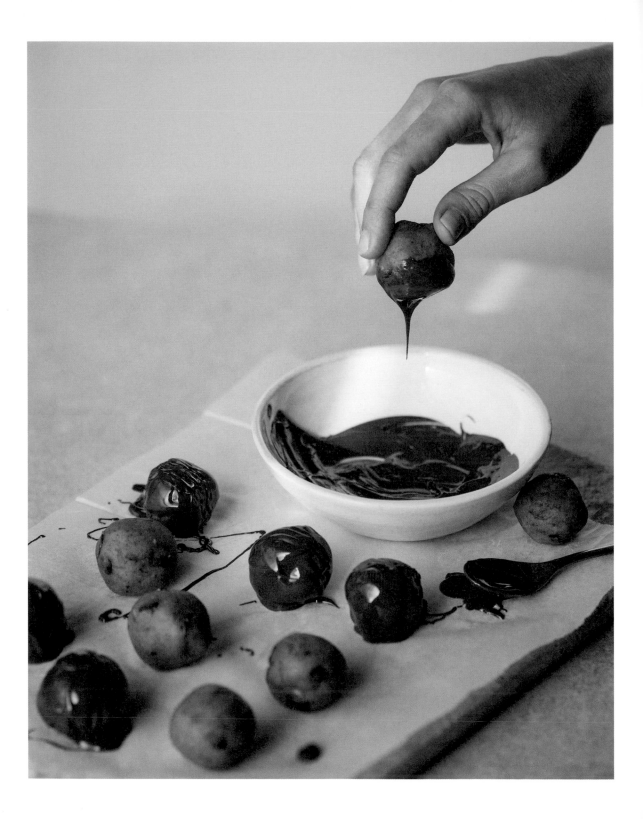

Prebiotic cookie dough drops

Makes **12 drops**   Prep **10 mins**

 Freezer

Raw cookie dough is full of nostalgic childhood memories of baking with my granny, so I wanted to recreate it with a version that I could also share with my gut microbes. This is a perfect afternoon pick-me-up, boasting 4.25 plant points in every ball, or an ideal treat for a movie night. Try it dotted into ice cream.

½ x 400g tin of chickpeas, drained and rinsed twice over

80g cashew butter (see below for a recipe), or nut or seed butter of choice

1 tsp vanilla extract

3 tbsp ground almonds

5 Medjool dates, pitted and roughly chopped (approx. 85g)

35g dark chocolate chips, roughly chopped

80g chocolate of choice for coating (optional)

Place the chickpeas, nut butter, vanilla extract, ground almonds and dates in a food processor and blitz for 1–2 minutes into a thick paste. Once ready, it usually makes a big ball of dough. If the mix is a little dry, add some water to help it blend (a bit at a time, up to 1 tbsp). Stir in the choc chips.

Split the dough into 12 even pieces and roll into balls. Place them on a tray lined with a piece of non-stick baking paper and chill in the fridge while you melt the chocolate (if using).

Break the chocolate into pieces and place in a heatproof mixing bowl. Melt by either placing over a saucepan of simmering water or heating in the microwave in 30-second bursts.

Decorate the drops with as much of the chocolate as you like – dunk fully, drizzle or pour a spoonful over. The cookie dough is also delicious on its own!

Homemade nut butter

(makes **a double batch, approx. 160g**)

Can't get your hands on cashew butter? Make your own!

Preheat the oven to 180°C/160°C fan/gas mark 4.

160g cashews

½ tbsp extra virgin olive oil

Place the cashews on a baking tray and bake for 5 minutes until they are golden and toasted. Remove from the oven and place in a food processor with the olive oil and sea salt. Blitz for a couple of minutes until a nut butter forms, scraping down the sides occasionally. As the cashews blend, they transform into a powder, then a clumpy mix and finally into a smooth butter.

Tip You can also try putting some of the cookie dough into the ice cream recipe on page 227. Just break it into pieces and stir through before freezing.

Storage The balls will keep for up to 1 week in the fridge, or in the freezer for up to 1 month.

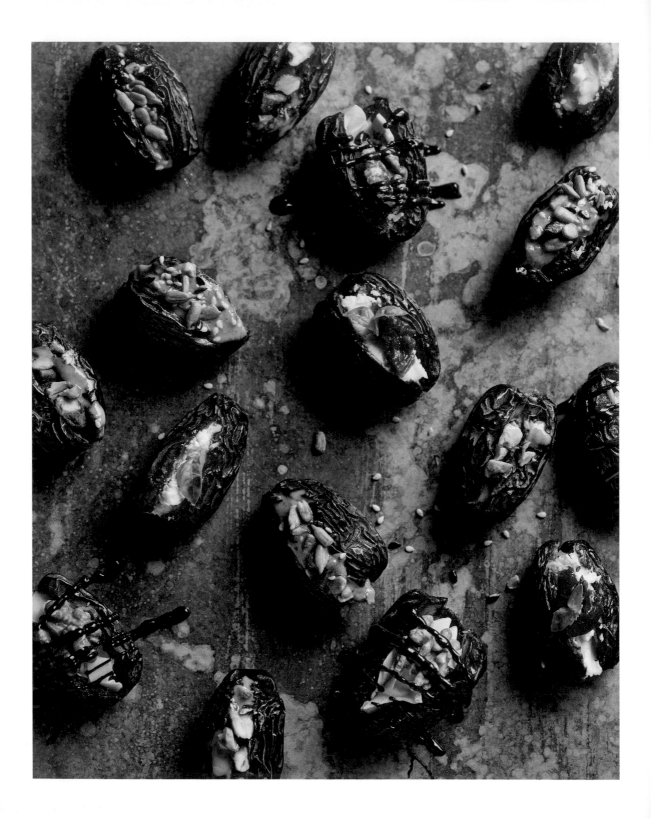

Stuffed dates – four ways

Plant Points
2.25

Serves **1**   Prep **2 mins**

 Freezer

I like to think of dates as nature's high-fibre sweeties, with their chewy sweetness giving that indulgent feel. They're my go-to for a quick treat, filled with my favourite combos of flavours. Feel free to experiment with your own stuffing ideas too. They're also great for freezing – if you have any left, that is!

1 pitted Medjool date and either:

a. Sweet and salty
10g goat's cheese
1 basil leaf
1 sundried tomato half, preserved in oil

b. Seed 'n' nut
1 heaped tsp nut butter of choice
a pinch of mixed seeds, toasted

c. Creamy tahini
1 heaped tsp tahini
5 pistachios

d. Choc nut
3g coconut flakes
1 walnut
a drizzle of melted dark chocolate

Slice the date lengthways, removing the pit to make a pocket.

Place your stuffing of choice in the pocket – it really is that simple!

Tip Pop your stuffed dates in the freezer for ready-to-go sweet treats all week – the freeze makes them even softer and creamier.

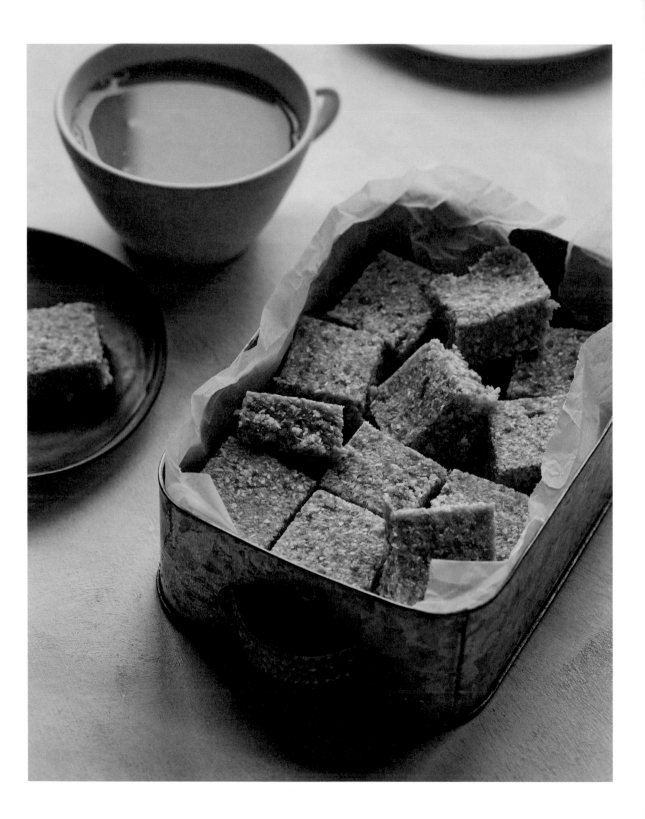

Four-ingredient citrus slice

Plant Points
3

Makes **25 squares**   Prep **10 mins, plus chilling time**

 Freezer

For those days when a piece of fruit won't cut it, but you're short on time for baking. Move over shop-bought muesli bars, this refreshing slice is the ultimate high-fibre accompaniment to a comforting cup of tea.

200g cashew nuts
200g desiccated coconut
150g dried apricots
juice of 1 large orange (approx. 80ml),
    plus zest to taste

Line the base and sides of an 18cm square brownie tin with non-stick baking paper.

Place the cashew nuts in a food processor and blitz for 30 seconds until ground. Add the coconut and apricots and pulse until the apricots are finely chopped. Add the orange juice, and blitz again until the mix forms a ball, this usually takes 1 minute or so. Taste, and add zest to preference.

Firmly press the mixture into the brownie tin with the back of a spoon. Chill in the fridge for 4 hours or until firm enough to cut. Slice into 25 squares.

Too impatient? Pop it in the freezer for 30 minutes before cutting with a sharp knife.

Storage These will keep in the fridge for up to 5 days. Or you can freeze the sliced squares between pieces of non-stick baking paper in an airtight container for up to 3 months.

Switch After an extra plant point? Add a grated carrot (approx. 70g prepped) and reduce the juice to 60ml.

Light bites

Garlicky aquafaba aioli

Makes **8 x 2 tbsp portions**   Prep **15 mins**

 FODMAP Lite   **Zero waste**

Like my grandad always used to say, 'Waste not want not.' After you've tried this thick and creamy aioli, you'll never look at the too-often-discarded liquid from tinned chickpeas the same way again. (Oh, and did you know the liquid contains prebiotics?) Not only is it easy to make, it's so versatile and goes with my smoky beet burgers (page 213), snack-o-clock veg fritters (page 179), popcorn chick-less nuggets (page 183) and just about everything else!

⅓ cup aquafaba from a tin of chickpeas (approx. 80ml), chilled
1 small garlic clove, grated or minced (approx. 2g)
a pinch of mustard powder
1½–2 tsp lemon juice, to taste
1 cup sunflower oil, or any neutral vegetable oil such as canola or avocado

Place everything, except the oil, in a jug and use a hand blender to blitz together for 1 minute.

Very slowly pour the oil into the jug while blending on fast speed. The mix will gradually thicken, taking 7–12 minutes to become thick and creamy. If you pour in the oil too fast, the mix won't thicken.

Adjust lemon and seasoning to taste.

Storage   Keep in the fridge in an airtight container for up to 2 weeks.

Creamy pistachio dip

Makes **8 portions (approx. 2 tbsp each)**   Prep **5 mins**

 Freezer

Don't let the name limit its true potential – this moreish combo is also delicious stirred through pasta like a creamy pesto, and it pairs perfectly with my foolproof fermented wheaten bread (page 176) as a spread. You'll be scraping out every last gram.

120g baby spinach leaves
1 small avocado, halved (approx. 110g prepped)
60g shelled pistachios
15g fresh basil
1 garlic clove (approx. 4 g)
juice of ½ 1 lemon (approx. 25–50ml), to taste
60ml extra virgin olive oil

Place all the ingredients in a food processor and blitz for approx. 1 minute if you like a little texture or 3 minutes if you prefer it smooth. Adjust lemon juice and seasoning to taste.

Storage   This will keep in the fridge for up to 1 week in an airtight container.

Tip   To prevent the avocado in the dip from browning, cover the dip in a thin layer of extra virgin olive oil or press a piece of cling film directly against the dip and store it in the fridge. Why does the browning happen? It's all thanks to a chemical reaction known as oxidation, where the air 'reacts' with those beneficial polyphenols, producing a compound called melanin – the pigment that makes our skin dark.

Smoky aubergine dip

Plant Points
6.25

Makes **7 portions (approx. 2 tbsp each)**   Prep **10 mins**   Cook **25 mins**

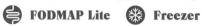 **FODMAP Lite**   **Freezer**

Creamy smoky aubergine – one of my favourite flavours, inspired by baba ghanoush. You can eat this with crunchy veg dipped in, spread on a seedy cracker (page 175) or wheaten bread (page 176), or as a side alongside some roasted veg and couscous. Did you know aubergine is a fruit? In fact, it's technically a large berry!

2 aubergines, halved lengthways
   (approx. 600g)
1 garlic clove
2 tbsp tahini
1 tbsp extra virgin olive oil
juice of 1 lemon (approx. 45ml),
   plus zest to taste
½ tsp cumin
½ tsp smoked paprika
2 tbsp capers, finely chopped (optional)

Toppers (optional):
1 tbsp parsley, finely chopped
   (approx. 2g)
2 tbsp pomegranate seeds
½ tsp sesame seeds

Preheat the grill and line a roasting tin with foil. Grease the foil with olive oil.

Place the aubergines skin up in the tin, and grill for 25 minutes or until the skin is fully charred. Add the garlic to roast for the final 5 minutes. Remove from the grill and leave until cool enough to handle.

Scoop out the flesh of the aubergines from the skin, and place in a high-powered blender along with the roasted garlic. Add the tahini, olive oil, lemon juice, spices, a pinch of sea salt and pepper, then blend until smooth.

Stir in the capers. Taste and adjust seasoning as needed.

Spoon into a bowl, and top with parsley, pomegranate or sesame seeds (if using).

Storage   This will keep in the fridge in an airtight container for 4–5 days.

No-added-sugar ketchup

Plant Points
6.5

Makes **15 portions (approx. 2 tbsp each)**   Prep **15 mins**   Cook **35 mins**

 FODMAP Lite   **Freezer**

Homemade ketchup packing that same flavour punch as the bottled stuff that many of us grew up on – but this one is full of diverse plant goodness without the added sugar. Perfect for dipping popcorn chick-less nuggets (page 183) into.

1 tsp extra virgin olive oil

1 small red onion, chopped (approx. 100g)

70g butternut squash, peeled and chopped

1 small red apple, chopped (approx. 100g)

1 carrot, chopped (approx. 70g)

½ tsp salt

1 x 400g tin of chopped tomatoes

1 tsp paprika

2 Medjool dates, pitted and roughly chopped (approx. 35g)

40g tomato puree

3 tbsp pickled beetroot juice, from the jar

Heat the olive oil in a saucepan. Add the onion, squash, apple, carrot and salt. Cover and cook over a low to moderate heat for 15 minutes until softened. If the mix starts to catch, add 1–2 tablespoons of cold water.

Add the tomatoes, paprika, dates and tomato puree. Turn the heat down to low and simmer for 20 minutes with the lid on.

Allow to cool before adding to a food processor, along with the beetroot juice. Blitz for 1 minute or until smooth, and adjust seasoning to taste.

Storage   This will keep in the fridge for 1 week or can be frozen for up to 1 month.

Tip   For some added microbes, add 1 tbsp of sauerkraut juice before blitzing. Transfer to an airtight container and leave out of direct sunlight for 4 hours (to allow the microbes to begin their fermenting feast). Taste and adjust seasoning as needed before storing in the fridge.

Switch   Prefer a smoky tomato sauce? Switch out the paprika for smoked paprika.

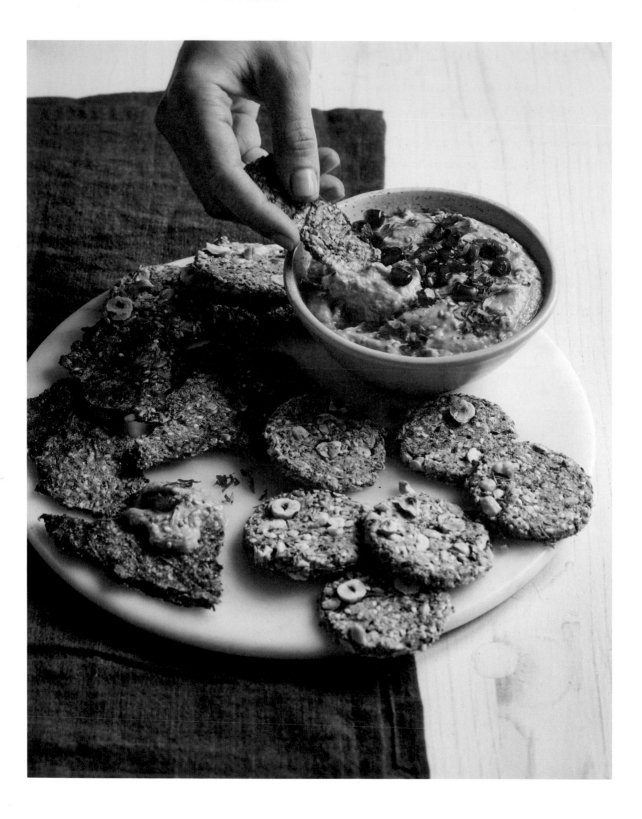

Plant Points
6.5

Seedy cracker duo

Serves **6 (approx. 3 crackers per portion)**   Prep **10 mins**   Cook **25 mins**

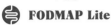 **FODMAP Lite**

A cupboard staple in my household. These crunchy crackers are the perfect delivery vehicle for a host of toppers when you need a quick bite between meals. They also serve up an impressive 4g of fibre per portion, which is more than four times as much as shop-bought cream crackers.

Base:
2 tbsp ground flaxseed
2 tbsp extra virgin olive oil
80g rye flour, or flour of choice
120g mixed seeds

Flavours (choose one):
Roasted hazelnut:
60g hazelnuts, chopped
1 tsp dried thyme

Cheesy beets:
20g raw beetroot, finely grated
2 tbsp nutritional yeast (approx. 10g)

Mix the flaxseed with 100ml boiling water and place to one side for 5 minutes to thicken.

Preheat the oven to *180˚C/160˚C fan/gas mark 4* and line a baking tray with non-stick baking paper.

If using grated beetroot, pat with paper towel to remove excess moisture.

Mix all the base ingredients, including the hydrated flaxseed and your chosen flavour (if using the hazelnuts, mix in only half of them, leaving the remainder to press on top) and a big pinch of sea salt, to form a rough dough. Leave for a few minutes to thicken.

Transfer the dough to a sheet of non-stick baking paper and place a second sheet over the top of the dough. Roll out the dough between the sheets of paper, as thin as you can get it. I roll mine paper-thin, for an extra-crispy cracker.

Sprinkle over a little extra sea salt to taste – and if using the hazelnuts, scatter the remaining nuts on top and gently press/roll into the dough.

Either cut out rounds with a 6cm cutter and place on the baking tray, or go for the rustic look and bake the biscuits in a whole sheet. Place in the oven and bake for 20–30 minutes, or until crispy and golden.

Place on a wire rack, and wait until completely cool before lifting them from the paper.

Storage These will keep in an airtight container at room temperature for up to 2 weeks if fully dried out.

Foolproof fermented wheaten bread

Plant Points
4.25

Makes **1 medium loaf (12 slices)**   Prep **10 mins (plus time for fermenting)**   Cook **40 mins**

❄️ **Freezer**

After I fell in love with wheaten bread in Ireland, my father-in-law entrusted me with his foolproof recipe. With a few gut-loving tweaks here and there, I present to you this game-changing recipe. Crunchy crusts with a deliciously moist and dense crumb – you'll never need to buy bread again.

300g wholemeal flour, plus extra
    for dusting
200g live thick yoghurt
½ tsp sea salt
1 tsp bicarbonate of soda
1 tbsp sesame seeds
1 tbsp pumpkin seeds
100g grated carrot (approx. 1
    large carrot)
3 sprigs thyme, leaves picked, or
    1 tsp dried thyme

Preheat the oven to *200˚C/180˚C fan/gas mark 6.*

Fermenting option:

Mix half the flour with the yoghurt and 100ml of water. Cover the bowl with a clean tea towel and leave to ferment for around 3 hours (keeping it out of direct sunlight). When you are ready to bake, mix in the remaining ingredients, using a butter knife to combine. Be careful not to overwork the dough as this will make it tough.

Non-fermenting option:

Combine all the ingredients, except for the yoghurt, in a large mixing bowl. Mix well. Add in the yoghurt along with 100ml of water, and stir with a butter knife to bring it together into a soft sticky dough. Be careful not to overwork the dough.

To bake:

Gently turn the dough on to a lightly floured baking tray and bring it together into a loaf shape. Score a cross on top with a sharp knife.

Bake for 40–50 minutes until golden, and check that the base is dry and the loaf sounds hollow when tapped. Place on a wire rack and let it cool completely.

Storage Well wrapped, it will keep for 2 days at room temperature, 5 days in the fridge, or up to 3 months in the freezer. I freeze mine in individual portions so I always have a serving of delicious bread on hand (just defrost in the microwave for a minute).

Switch If you've already had carrots this week, the recipe also works with 100g courgette, just reduce the water to 80ml.

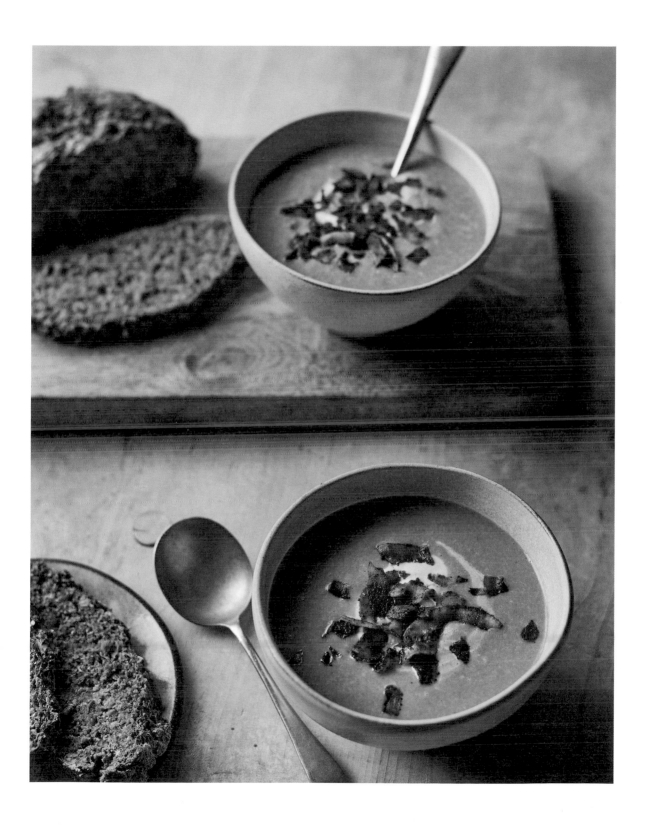

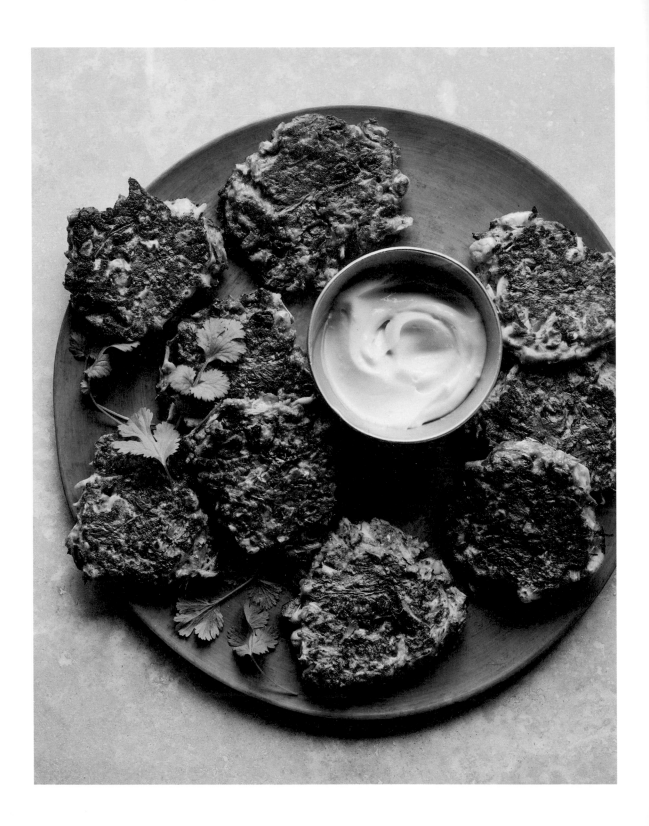

Snack-o-clock veg fritters

Plant Points 5.5

Makes **10 fritters**   Prep **10 mins**   Cook **20 mins**

FODMAP Lite   **Fridge raid**

Perfect for packing in your plant points and using up any leftover veg in your fridge. I love pairing these with my garlicky aquafaba aioli (page 170), or adding a side salad and some sweet potato wedges for a flavourful feast!

3 large eggs
80g broad beans, fresh or tinned
300g stir-fry mixed veg (e.g. shredded
    cabbage, carrots, onion)
60g wholemeal flour, or flour of choice
2 tbsp red miso
2 tbsp extra virgin olive oil, for frying
10g fresh coriander leaves

Blitz the eggs in a food processor for 12 seconds or so until they are nice and fluffy. Add in the broad beans and mixed veg and blend for a few seconds to roughly break up the beans and any larger pieces of veg.

Transfer to a large mixing bowl. Add the flour, miso and pepper to taste. Mix to form a thick batter.

Heat a shallow layer of olive oil in a large frying pan. Once the pan is hot, add 60g (¼ cup) of the batter into the pan for each fritter. Press a few coriander leaves on to the surface of the batter.

Fry for 5–6 minutes over a medium heat with the lid on until golden brown, then flip and cook for a further 1–2 minutes on the other side. Repeat until you've used all the batter. They are delicate to start off with, so try not to peep at the bottom of the fritters for the first couple of minutes until they have started to crisp up.

Once cooked, serve and enjoy while warm – or put them in your lunchbox for the next day!

Tip You can experiment with other miso such as white miso and you'll end up with a different-tasting fritter. White miso is sweeter, yellow miso is earthy, red miso is packed with umami, yum!

Storage Leftover fritters can be kept in the fridge for 3 days.

Switch After an extra plant point? Add in 100g corn kernels and reduce the stir-fry mix to 200g.

All-the-greens filo swirl

Serves **4**   Prep **20 mins**   Cook **25 mins**

 FODMAP Lite   **Freezer**

Inspired by the Greek spanakopita I love so much, this version packs in loads of veg and flavour. It's an ideal centrepiece for lunch with friends, and also makes a great sausage roll substitute for picnics and hungry kids. Offering 6g of fibre per portion, you won't mind the kids coming back for seconds.

150g spring greens, roughly chopped
50g spinach, finely chopped
100g peas, fresh or frozen
80g green beans, diced
250g ricotta
200g feta, crumbled
10g dill, roughly chopped
6 sheets of filo pastry, fresh
1 tbsp sesame seeds
extra virgin olive oil, for brushing

Preheat the oven to *220°C/200°C fan/gas mark 7*.

Start by wilting the spring greens and spinach – either in a large saucepan with a splash of water over a medium heat, or in the microwave for 3 minutes. Allow to cool then, using clean hands, squeeze out any excess moisture and transfer to a large mixing bowl.

Add the peas, beans, ricotta, feta and dill, and mix well to combine. Season to taste.

Take a sheet of filo and lay it out on the worktop (landscape). Brush a little oil down one short edge and attach another sheet. Repeat so you have one long strip of 3 sheets of filo. Now brush oil all over it and lay 3 additional sheets on top, so you have a double thickness.

Spread the filling out in a long line down the edge closest to you, leaving a 2cm border. Then, start to tightly roll, and keep rolling until you have one long tube. Brush the top with olive oil.

If you are making the swirl, take one end and gently roll it in on itself. Continue with the whole roll until you have a large spiral pie. Alternatively, you can cut into lengths like sausage rolls – perfect for picnics and taking with you on-the-go.

Transfer to a lined baking tray and sprinkle with the sesame seeds. Bake in the oven for 25–30 minutes until the filo is golden and crisp.

Best straight out of the oven.

Storage Leftovers can be kept in the fridge for up to 3 days. If you'd prefer to prep in adavance, it can be kept in the freezer for up to 1 month (if using fresh filo) – just add 5–10 minutes to the cooking time.

Tip You need to work fast with the filo, otherwise it will dry out. Brush with oil if it becomes too dry to roll.

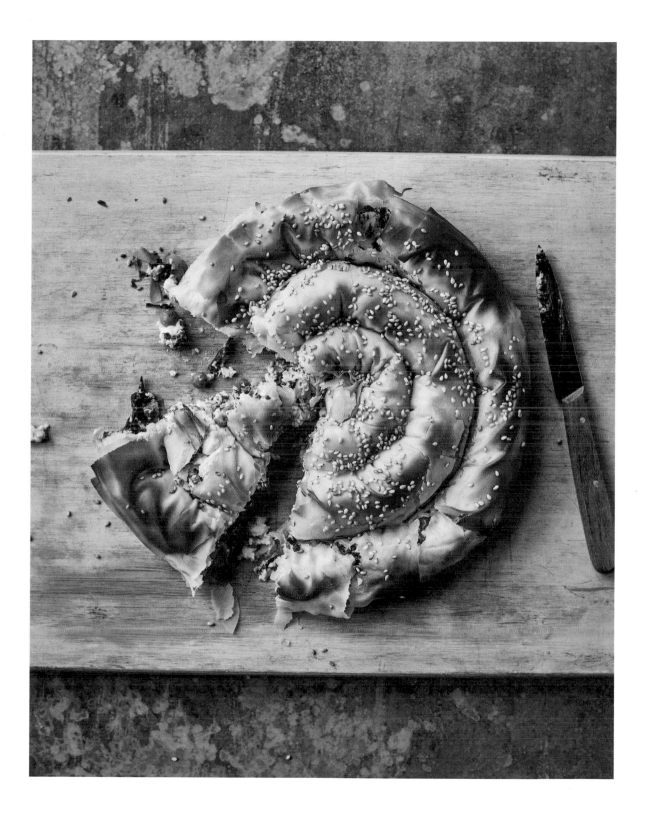

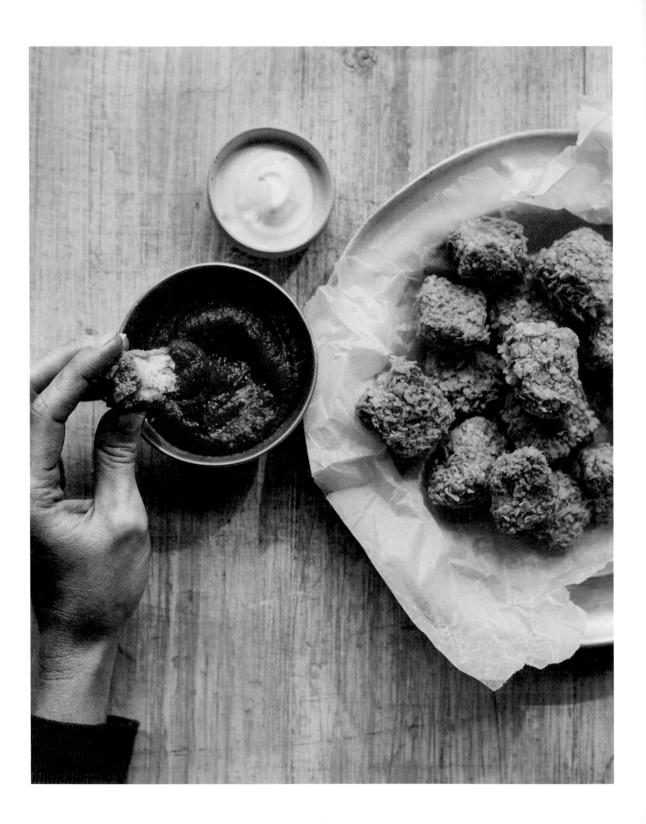

Popcorn chick-less nuggets

Makes **16 nuggets**   Prep **10 mins**   Cook **15 mins**

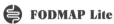 **FODMAP Lite**

Are you a sucker for ultra-processed chicken nuggets? I used to be too! But then I discovered these equally crispy and juicy plant-based alternatives. Take each mouthful to the next level with a dip of garlicky aquafaba aioli (page 170) or no-added-sugar ketchup (page 173).

280g extra-firm tofu
60g wholemeal flour, or flour of choice
100ml soy milk, or milk of choice
½ tsp smoked paprika
2 tbsp nutritional yeast (approx. 10g)
   (optional)
80g cornflakes, crushed

Preheat the oven to *200°C/180°C fan/gas mark 6.*

Cut the tofu into 3cm x 3cm x 2cm nuggets.

In a large bowl, mix the flour, milk, paprika, a big pinch of sea salt and the nutritional yeast (if using). Stir to form a thick batter.

Place the crushed cornflakes in a separate bowl.

Dip each tofu nugget into the batter, shaking off any excess, before rolling it in the crushed cornflakes. Place on a baking tray lined with non-stick baking paper. Once all of the nuggets are coated, pop in the oven for 15 minutes or until golden and crispy.

Best enjoyed straight out of the oven with aioli, ketchup or a mix of both!

Switch Get experimental with your herbs and spices; instead of the paprika try mixed herbs, cumin or thyme.

Courgette and hazelnut salad

Serves **2**   Prep **10 mins**   Cook **5 mins**

 FODMAP Lite

When you and your microbes are craving something light and refreshing that doesn't fall short on either the plant points or the flavour front, look no further. This light bite will really hit the spot, giving you 7g of fibre and getting you 9.5 plant points closer to your weekly target.

30g hazelnuts
20g mixed seeds
2 courgettes (approx. 400g)
40g mixed salad leaves (e.g. spinach, rocket, watercress)
60g feta, crumbled

Dressing:
1 tbsp extra virgin olive oil
juice of ½ orange (approx. 40ml), plus zest to taste
2 tsp cider vinegar of choice
1 tsp honey

Toppers:
2 tsp mint leaves, finely chopped
40g pomegranate seeds

Preheat the oven to *180˚C/160˚C/gas mark 4*.

Spread the hazelnuts out on a baking tray and bake for 5 minutes until golden, adding the seeds to the tray for the final 2 minutes. Set aside to cool, then roughly chop the hazelnuts.

Combine the dressing ingredients. Season and adjust flavours to taste.

In a small bowl, peel the courgettes into ribbons (using a potato peeler) before pouring the dressing on top. Allow to marinate for a few minutes before tossing in the salad leaves.

Divide the courgette mix between two serving bowls, followed by the feta, hazelnuts and seeds.

Pour any leftover dressing on top before scattering the mint leaves and pomegranate seeds (if using) on top.

Tip Want to turn this into a main meal? It goes perfectly with a grilled fillet of white fish and a side of toasted sourdough.

Leafy taco wraps

Serves **2**   Prep **10 mins**

A flavour-filled bean mix nestled in a crisp lettuce cup, for a light bite or lunch on-the-go, this wrap feeds your gut 16g of fibre too (that's more than half your daily needs!). Want a heartier option to transform your Taco Tuesdays? Swap the lettuce for wholemeal tortillas.

1 cob of sweetcorn, raw, or 100g tinned corn
1 x 400g tin of black-eyed peas, drained and rinsed
100g fresh salsa
1 small avocado, diced (approx. 110g prepped)
2 roasted red peppers from the jar, roughly chopped (approx. 100g)
30g feta, chopped into 1cm cubes
¼ tsp cumin

To serve (optional):
4 large lettuce leaves of choice
5g fresh coriander
¼ cup live thick yoghurt
1 fresh chilli, sliced
½ lime, cut into wedges

Cut the corn off the cob and add to a mixing bowl, along with the other base ingredients. Toss to combine and season to taste.

To serve, lay out the lettuce leaves. Place a large spoonful of the bean mix on each leaf, followed by the coriander, yoghurt, chilli and lime (if using).

Roll up the lettuce wraps and dig in.

Switch   Can't get your hands on black-eyed peas? Use tinned black beans, adzuki or kidney beans instead. You can also swap the roasted red pepper for fresh bell pepper.

Storage   The bean mix will keep in the fridge for 3 days. See the tip at the bottom of page 171 to prevent the avocado from browning. But remember, even if it does go brown, it's still perfectly good to eat!

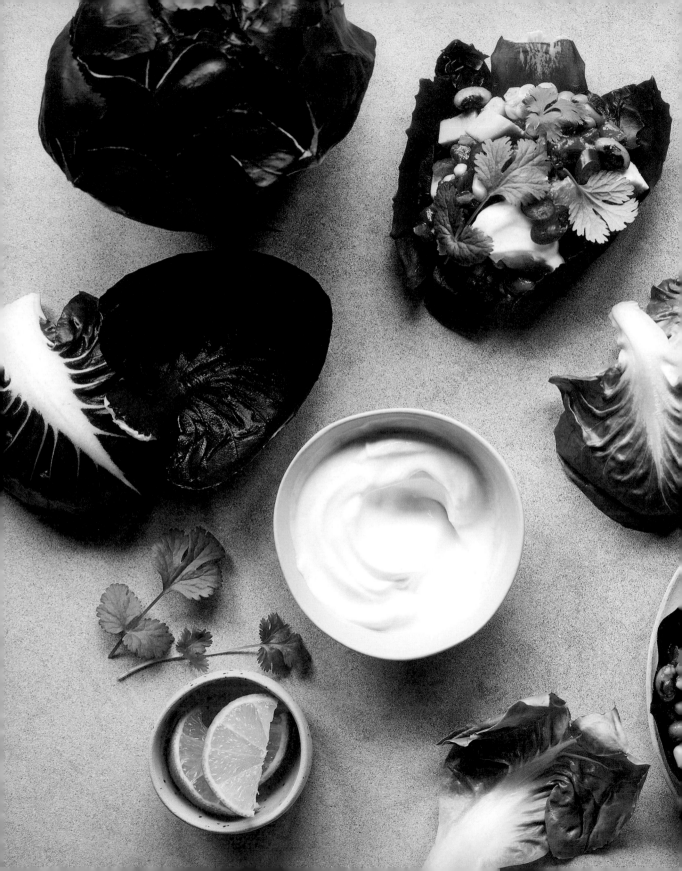

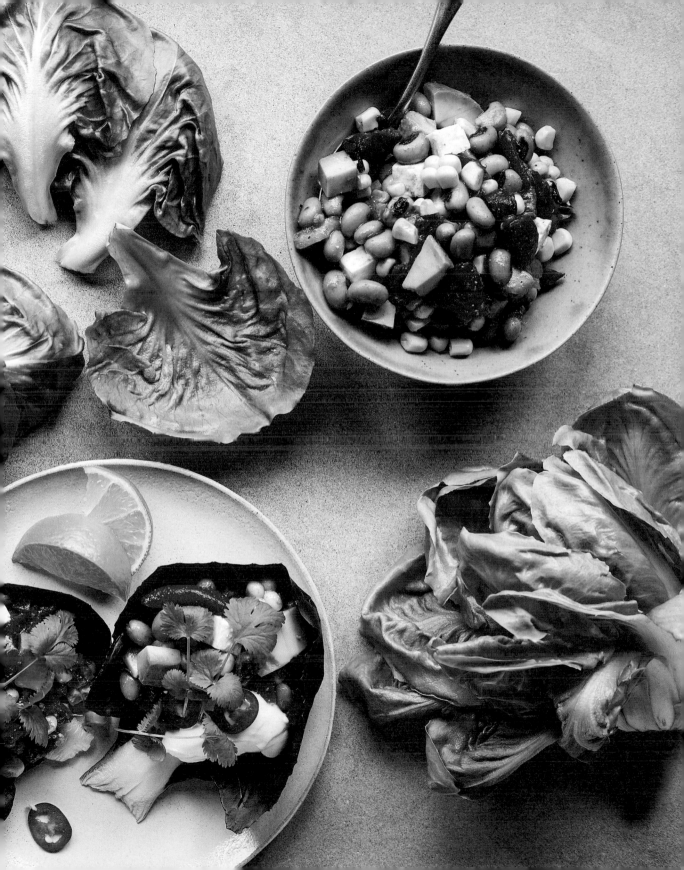

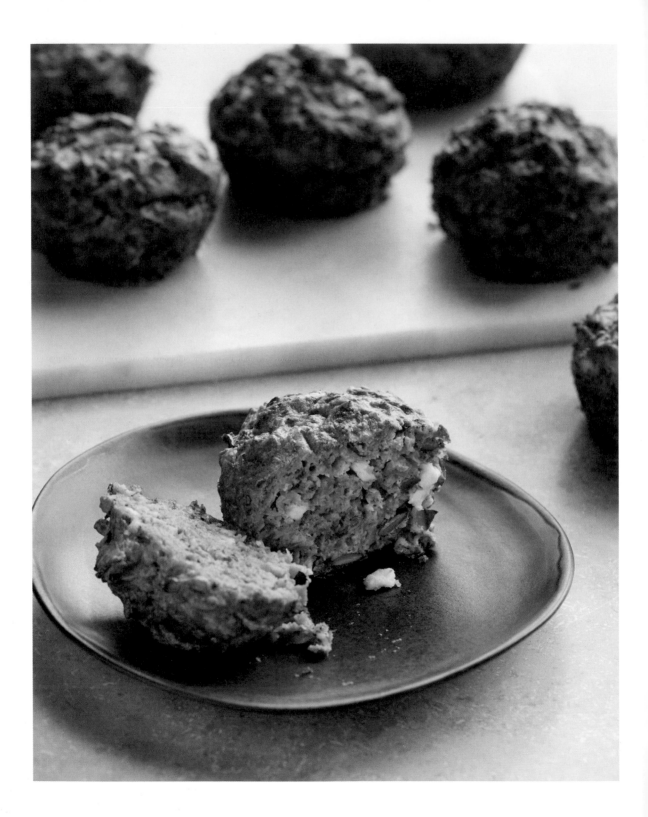

Butternut muffins

Makes **12 muffins**   Prep **15 mins**   Cook **30 mins**

 FODMAP Lite   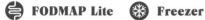 **Freezer**

These savoury, moist muffins are ideal to make in bulk and then freeze, so you always have something tasty and nourishing ready to go when hunger strikes. Great for lunchboxes or as an afternoon snack.

300g butternut squash, grated
1 courgette, grated (approx. 150g prepped)
160g spelt flour, or flour of choice
2 tsp baking powder
4 large eggs, beaten
3 tbsp extra virgin olive oil
100g feta, crumbled
3 tbsp mixed seeds (approx. 30g)
10g fresh basil, finely chopped
1 tsp chilli flakes (optional)
2 tsp smoked paprika
½ tsp salt, or to preference

Preheat the oven to *200°C/180°C fan/gas mark 6*. Grease a 12-hole muffin tin and add a disc of non-stick baking paper to the bottom of each hole to prevent sticking.

Place the grated squash and courgette in a large mixing bowl. Add the flour and baking powder and stir to coat the veg.

Add the eggs and the oil, and stir well to incorporate evenly.

Finally, add the feta, seeds, basil, chilli flakes (if using), paprika and salt, and stir well. You should have a thick batter. If it's a little dry, add a splash of your choice of milk.

Fill each hole in the muffin tin to just below the top, allowing room for them to rise. Place the tin in the oven for around 30–35 minutes (or until a skewer comes out clean). Place on a wire rack to cool.

These muffins are delicious when eaten still warm, or cold the next day.

Storage Will keep in the fridge for 3 days in an airtight container. You can also freeze them for up to 2 months, and defrost in the microwave when hunger strikes.

Tip For an extra plant point, add in 50g of frozen peas.

Switch If squash isn't in season, use sweet potato instead.

Packed lunches

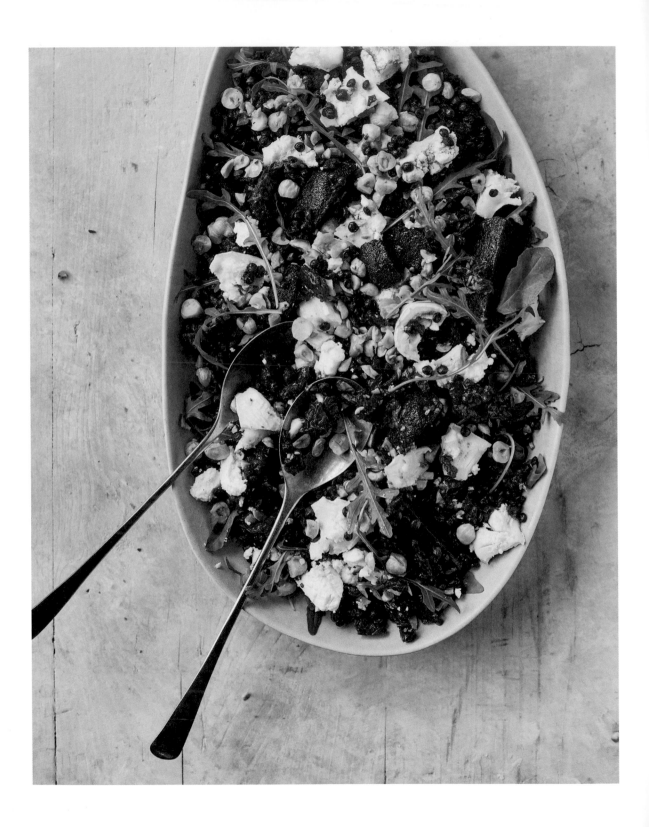

Beetroot, lentil and goat's cheese salad

Plant Points
5.25

Serves **4**   Prep **10 mins**   Cook **5 mins**

Because boring salads have no place on my plate! This winning combo features layers of earthy flavours rounded off with creamy goat's cheese, and will give you a whopping 14g of fibre per portion. It might even have you making a double batch next time round.

2 x 250g pouch of cooked Puy lentils
4 large cooked beetroots, cut into
   wedges
20 sundried tomato halves, preserved in
   oil, roughly chopped

Dressing:
2 tbsp balsamic vinegar
1 tsp honey, or sweetener of choice
2 tbsp extra virgin olive oil

Toppers:
60g leaves of choice (e.g. spinach,
   rocket, watercress)
160g goat's cheese, crumbled
60g hazelnuts, roughly chopped

Add the lentils, beetroot and sundried tomatoes to a mixing bowl.

Whisk together the dressing ingredients before pouring over the lentils and veg in the bowl. Let the dressing marinate the ingredients for at least 5 minutes (ideally 30 minutes if you have the time) while you prep the toppers.

Preheat the oven to *180˚C/160˚C fan/gas mark 4.*

Place the blanched hazelnuts on a baking tray and bake for 5 minutes until golden. Set aside to cool, then chop roughly

For lunch on the go, first add the marinated mix to a glass jar, followed by the goat's cheese, hazelnuts and leaves to prevent them getting soggy. Give it a good stir before digging in.

Alternatively, for a leisurely lunch, on a large serving tray plate the green leaves, followed by the marinated mix. Top with goat's cheese and the hazelnuts. Toss before serving – yum!

Storage   The marinated mix will keep for up to 3 days in the fridge. The salad also keeps in the fridge for up to 3 days, but the leaves are best added fresh as you serve to prevent them going soggy.

Roasted veg and freekeh salad

Serves **4**   Prep **10 mins**   Cook **25 mins**

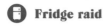 **Fridge raid**

A hearty Middle Eastern-inspired salad, full of flavour and designed to keep you fibre-fuelled past the 3 p.m. slump. I love a combination of peppers, courgettes, red onion, green beans, cherry tomatoes, cauliflower and fresh corn from the cob, but any of your favourites or leftovers will work too.

800g mixed veg (I love ready-to-roast, Mediterranean-style veg), roughly chopped
2 tbsp extra virgin olive oil
1 tbsp harissa, or more to taste
2 x 250g pouch cooked freekeh (or 250g raw), or wholegrains of choice
2 tbsp mixed seeds
20g pecans, or nut of choice
40g salad leaves

Toppers (optional):
¼ cup live thick yoghurt
2 tsp harissa
fresh parsley leaves (approx. 5g)

Preheat the oven to *200°C/180°C fan/gas mark 6.*

Place your choice of mixed veg in a large roasting tin. Stir the oil and harissa together before drizzling over them and season to taste. Using your hands, mix everything together before placing in the oven to cook for 15 minutes.

Cook the freekeh according to packet instructions (2 minutes for precooked; approx. 20 minutes in boiling water for raw).

Remove from the oven and turn the veg. Scatter the mixed seeds and pecans on top and then return to the oven for another 10 minutes, or until golden brown.

Add the cooled freekeh to a mixing bowl along with the salad leaves and the roast veg, and toss to combine.

For the toppers, combine the yoghurt and harissa (if using), before dolloping on top of the plated veg along with the parsley.

Tip Any time you're having roast veg, make a double batch to use for this dish.

Smoked mackerel, new potato and apple salad

Serves **4**   Prep **10 mins**   Cook **15 mins**

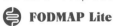 **FODMAP Lite**

Don't be deceived by its simplicity, this salad oozes flavour. Delicious warm or cold, there's something extra-special about the delicate smoked fish, crunchy apple and tender veg, wrapped in a creamy dressing with a subtle tang from the mustard. It's also a good source of fibre, including resistant starch from the chilled potatoes, and omega-3.

12 baby new potatoes, halved
200g asparagus spears, trimmed
60g cashews, raw
2 apples, cored and sliced
2 fennel bulbs, sliced
80g mixed salad leaves
320g smoked mackerel

Dressing:
¼ cup live thick yoghurt
2 tsp Dijon mustard
juice of 1 lemon (approx. 45ml)
5–10g fresh dill, chopped, to taste
a grind of black pepper

Preheat the oven to *180°C/160°C fan/gas mark 4*.

Boil the potatoes in a saucepan, along with a pinch of salt, for 15 minutes (or until tender).

Add the asparagus spears to the potatoes for the last 3 minutes of cooking, then drain everything and put to one side to cool slightly.

While the potatoes are cooking, place the cashews on a baking tray and bake for 5 minutes or until golden. Remove from the oven and set aside to cool.

In a large mixing bowl whisk together all the dressing ingredients. Then add all the base ingredients, except for the salad leaves to prevent them getting soggy (apple, fennel and potatoes).

Once you are ready to enjoy, toss in the salad leaves and season to taste.

Switch Not into mackerel? Switch out for your fish of choice, an egg, or legumes such as butter beans.

Storage Keeps in the fridge for up to 3 days, but leaves are best added fresh as you serve to prevent them wilting.

Sweet jacket potato trio

Don't underestimate the versatility of sweet potato. Sweet, savoury, hot or cold, this trio can flex around your mood. Creamy flavour aside, they're also a nourishing source of fibre and are loaded with beta-carotene, one of those phytochemicals with impressive antioxidant powers . . . And we haven't even touched on the toppers yet, which together deliver at least a third of your daily fibre needs.

Sweet jacket potato with black beans

Plant Points 5.25

Serves **2**   Prep **5 mins**   Cook **10/50 mins**

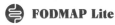 **FODMAP Lite**

2 sweet potatoes (approx. 180g each)
½ tbsp extra virgin olive oil
1 garlic clove, grated or crushed (approx. 4g)
1 x 400g tin of black beans, drained and rinsed
80g fresh spinach
¼ tsp cayenne pepper

Toppers:
2 tbsp live thick yoghurt
½ avocado, sliced (approx. 80g)
2 pickled chillis or jalapeños
coriander leaves
lime wedges (optional)

The sweet jacket potato

Prick the sweet potatoes with a fork (this helps prevent the skin from splitting) before cooking them – either in the microwave with a splash of water for 8–10 minutes (or until tender all the way through), or by baking in the oven for 50 minutes at *200°C/180°C fan/gas mark 6*. While the potatoes are cooking start making the filling.

The filling

Heat the olive oil in a saucepan and add the garlic. Cook for 1 minute. Add the black beans and cook for a further few minutes to heat the beans all the way through before stirring in the spinach and cayenne pepper. Pop a lid on the saucepan for 2 minutes, as the steam will help the spinach to wilt, then stir. Taste and adjust cayenne pepper, and season to preference.

Cut each sweet potato in half and fill with the black bean mix. Top with the yoghurt, avocado (if you're taking this for lunch you might prefer to do this just before eating, to stop it browning), a pickled chilli, some fresh coriander leaves and a squeeze of lime juice (if using). Season to taste.

Storage Keeps in the fridge for up to 3 days.

Switch Already had black beans this week? Switch out for pinto beans.

Tip Cook extra sweet potato and make the one-minute sweet potato slider on page 302.

Sweet jacket potato with nut-free pesto

Plant Points 5

Serves **2**   Prep **15 mins**   Cook **10/50 mins**

 FODMAP Lite   **Freezer**

2 sweet potatoes (approx. 180g each)

1 tsp extra virgin olive oil

1 x 400g tin of butter beans, drained and rinsed

1 tsp za'atar

Pesto (makes 150g):

40g Parmesan, grated

1 small garlic clove (approx. 3g)

40g pumpkin seeds, toasted

30g fresh basil

60ml extra virgin olive oil

juice of ½ lemon (approx. 25ml)

Toppers (optional):

extra basil leaves

cherry tomatoes, halved

Prepare and cook the potato in the same way as on page 196.

Heat the oil in a medium frying pan. Add the butter beans and za'atar, and cook for a further few minutes to heat the beans all the way through. Remove from the heat and season to taste.

To a food processor add all the pesto ingredients and pulse until you have a textured green paste. Season to taste.

Cut the potatoes in half and top with the butter bean mix, 4 tablespoons of pesto, tomatoes and a few basil leaves.

Storage Any leftover pesto can be kept in fridge for up to 1 week. Cover the surface with either a drizzle of olive oil or cling film. Or you can freeze it for up to 3 months.

PB & J sweet jacket potato

Plant Points 8.25

Serves **2**   Prep **10 mins**   Cook **15/50 mins**

 FODMAP Lite   **Freezer**

2 sweet potatoes (approx. 180g each)

1 banana, peeled (approx. 100g)

a sprinkle of cinnamon

2 tbsp nut butter of choice

Chia berry jam (makes 200g):

250g frozen raspberries

juice of ½ orange (approx. 40ml)

2 tbsp chia seeds

honey or sweetener of choice, to taste

Topper:

2 tsp flaked coconut or mixed seeds, toasted (optional)

Prepare and cook the potato in the same way as on page 196.

To make the jam, place the raspberries and orange juice in a small saucepan over a medium heat, and simmer for 5–7 minutes until the berries have broken down and the liquid has reduced. Remove from the heat, stir in the seeds, and leave to stand for a few minutes until thickened. Sweeten to taste.

While you're waiting for the jam to thicken, slice the banana and sprinkle with cinnamon. Heat a small frying pan over a medium heat. Add the banana and cook for 30 seconds on each side, or until caramelized.

Cut the potatoes in half and add the banana, 2 tbsp of chia jam per potato, a drizzle of nut butter, and coconut or seeds (if using).

Storage The jam will keep in the fridge for up to 1 week in an airtight container, or can be frozen for up to 3 months.

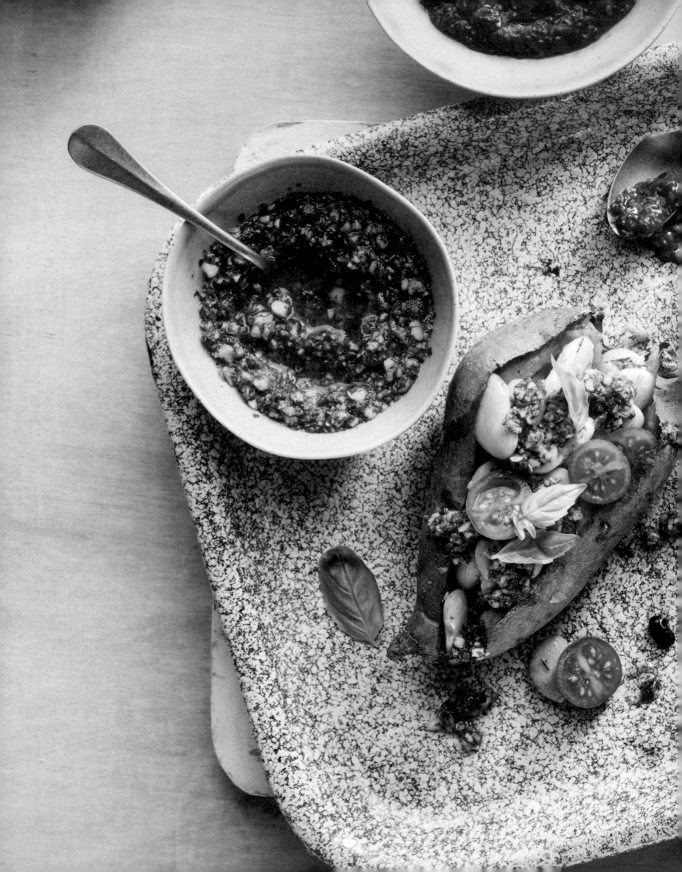

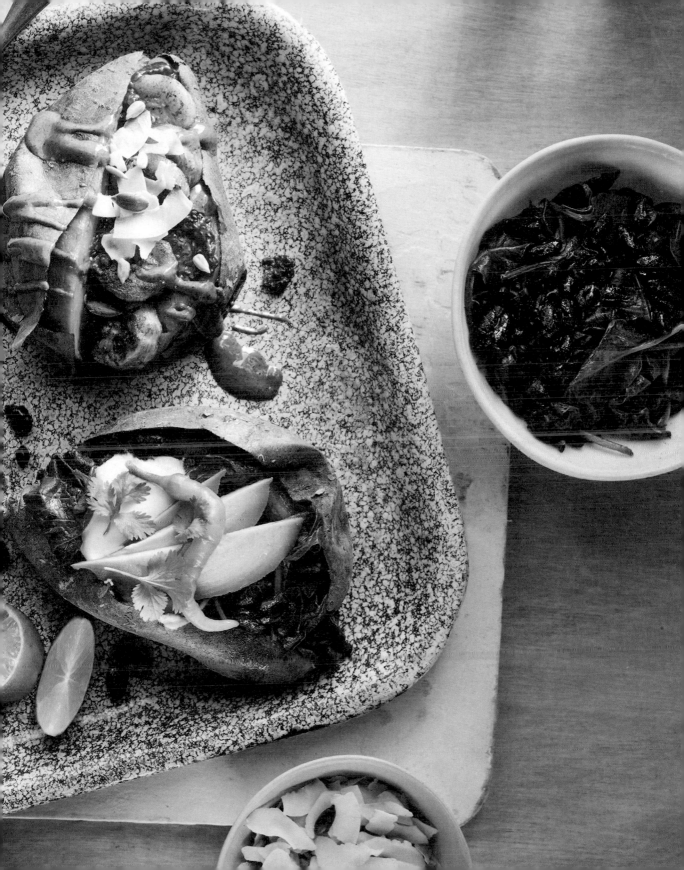

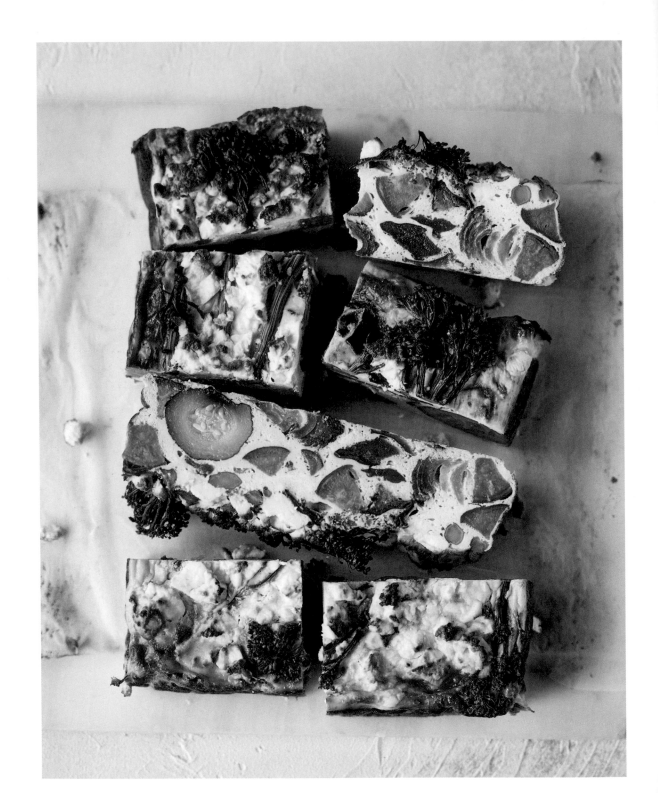

Chunky veg and feta frittata

Plant Points
6.75

Serves **8**   Prep **15 mins**   Cook **1 hour 20 mins**

⊜ **FODMAP Lite**   🄵 **Fridge raid**

Hot or cold, for breakfast, lunch or dinner – things don't get much more versatile than this fibre-filled frittata. Mix up the veg to keep it seasonal and interesting for endless weekday options. It's earned a regular spot on my menu.

1 red onion (approx. 180g), cut into
    8 wedges

1 courgette (approx. 200g), cut into
    4 long quarters

1 aubergine (approx. 400g), cut into
    8 long strips

1 red pepper (approx. 150g), cut into
    6 long strips

2 sweet potatoes (approx. 300g), each
    cut into 6 long strips

4 sprigs thyme, leaves picked, or
    1 tsp dried thyme

2 tsp chilli flakes (optional)

10 large eggs

50g extra virgin olive oil, plus more
    for drizzling

200g full-fat Greek yoghurt

8 pieces Tenderstem broccoli

200g feta, crumbled

Preheat the oven to *200˚C/180˚C fan/gas mark 6*.

Line a large baking tray with non-stick baking paper. Add in all the veg except for the broccoli (onion, courgette, aubergine, red pepper and sweet potato). Mix with the thyme leaves, a generous drizzle of olive oil, a big pinch of sea salt and chilli (if using), and roast for 30 minutes.

Line the base and sides of a deep 25cm square cake tin. Layer the roasted veg into the tin, alternating the different types. This will ensure that each slice of frittata has a selection of veg when cut, as pictured on page 200.

Stir together the eggs, olive oil and yoghurt until just combined, along with a big pinch of salt and a grind of pepper – you don't want to add too much air into the egg. Pour this mix over the veg, then add the broccoli and sprinkle the feta on top.

Reduce oven temperature to *180˚C/160˚C fan/gas mark 4*. Bake for 50–60 minutes, or until the middle has just set. If the top starts to brown earlier, cover with foil. Why not take some time out for yourself while it's cooking?

How do you know when the frittata is done? The centre should be no longer jiggly. For extra reassurance, using a sharp knife, cut into the centre of the frittata. If raw egg runs into the cut, it needs a little longer in the oven.

Let cool for at least 10 minutes, then slice to serve.

Tip You can use live yoghurt instead of full-fat Greek here – the microbes die off in high temperatures, so there is no extra benefit to using it in this recipe, but there's also no downside!

Storage Will keep in the fridge for up to 3 days.

Tofu fried wholegrains with crunchy cashews

Serves **2** Prep **15 mins** Cook **10 mins (or 25 mins if cooking wholegrains)**

 FODMAP Lite   **Fridge raid**

It's easy to get stuck in a wholegrain rut, eating the same types on repeat. This deliciously diverse take on a classic fried rice dish is here to show you that there are so many amazing textures and flavours in the world of wholegrains. Plus, it doesn't just deliver on flavour, but fibre (11g) and plant points (12.5) too, delivering a third of your daily and weekly goals respectively.

250g precooked mixed wholegrains pouch, or 100g raw wholegrains
40g cashews
2 tsp sesame oil
2 garlic cloves, grated or minced
10g fresh ginger, peeled and grated
1 large red chilli, finely chopped (approx. 20g) (optional)
200g mixed stir-fry veg (e.g. cabbage, carrots, peppers, red onion)
50g beansprouts (optional)
50g peas, fresh or frozen
1 tbsp soy sauce, more to taste
1 spring onion, sliced (approx. 10g)

Tofu scramble:
1 tsp sesame oil
150g silken tofu
¼ tsp turmeric
¼ tsp paprika
1 tbsp nutritional yeast (approx. 5g) (optional)
¼ tsp black pepper

If you're cooking your own wholegrains, cook those first to the packet instructions. You can buy ready-mixed quick-cook wholegrains that are usually ready in 10 minutes.

Heat a large frying pan over a medium heat. Add the cashews and toast for a few minutes, stirring frequently. Tip on to a plate and set aside.

Start your tofu scramble by heating 1 tsp sesame oil in the same pan. Crumble in the tofu with your hands, then add the turmeric, paprika, nutritional yeast and black pepper. Cook for 3–4 minutes until any liquid has reduced. Tip on to a plate and set aside.

To the same pan, add another teaspoon of sesame oil along with the garlic, ginger and chilli (if using) and cook for 1 minute. Add the stir-fry veg and the beansprouts (if using). Cook for 3–4 minutes, so they still have a little crunch to them.

Finally, stir in the remaining ingredients (wholegrains, soy sauce, spring onions and tofu scramble) and cook for 1–2 minutes to heat through.

Taste and adjust seasoning to preference, then serve topped with the toasted cashews.

Tip You can always switch out the tofu scramble for two large eggs, scrambled, with the turmeric and black pepper.

Storage Keeps in the fridge for up to 3 days.

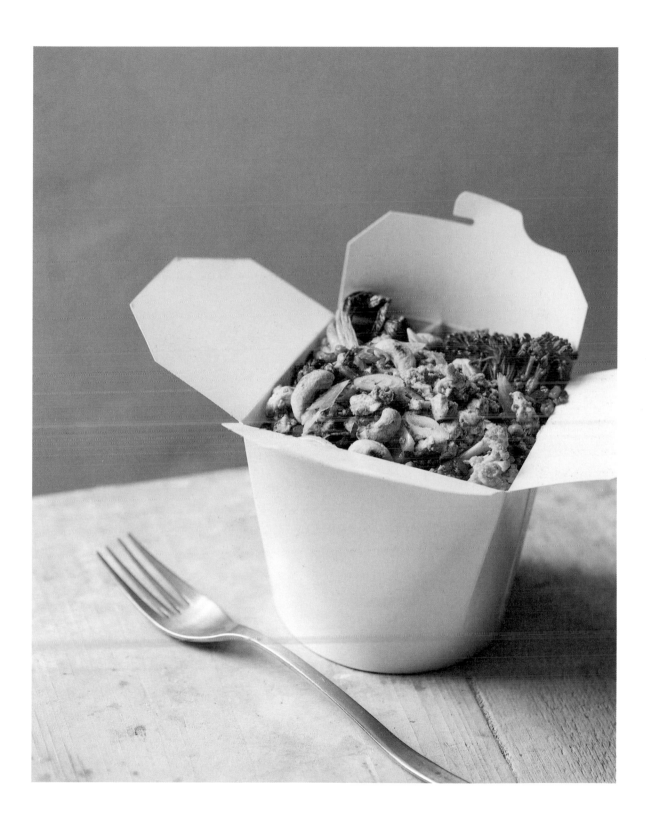

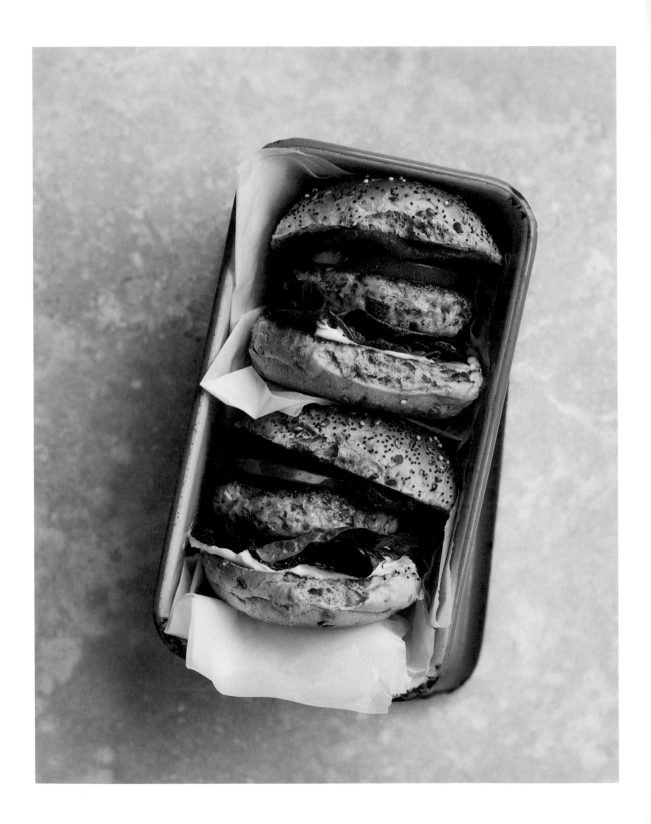

Reinvented chicken burger

Serves **2**   Prep **5 mins**   Cook **10 mins**

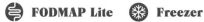 **FODMAP Lite**   ✳ **Freezer**

Left overnight for the flavours to really infuse, this burger mix is even better the second time round. Pair with crispy lettuce, juicy tomato and beetroot, and top with a dollop of creamy aioli and ketchup for the ultimate burger.

½ tbsp extra virgin olive oil
230g chicken 'n' veg meaty ball mix
   (see page 256)

Toppers:
2 seedy burger buns
2 large lettuce leaves
1 large tomato, sliced
4 slices of pickled beetroot
   (approx. 50g)
garlicky aquafaba aioli (page 170)
no-sugar-added ketchup (page 173)

Using clean hands, shape the chicken mix into two evenly sized burgers. The mixture will feel wet, but don't be tempted to add extra breadcrumbs; it will be nice and juicy when cooked.

Heat the olive oil in a frying pan on a medium-high heat, and cook the burgers for 5–6 minutes each side until they are golden brown on the outside and cooked through.

Slice your burger buns (you can also toast them if you like), then layer up the lettuce, tomato, beetroot, aioli and ketchup to make a classic burger – or add whatever else you like! Some of my favourites include grilled onions, a fried egg, avocado and portobello mushrooms.

Storage Once cooked, the burgers can be frozen for up to 1 month.

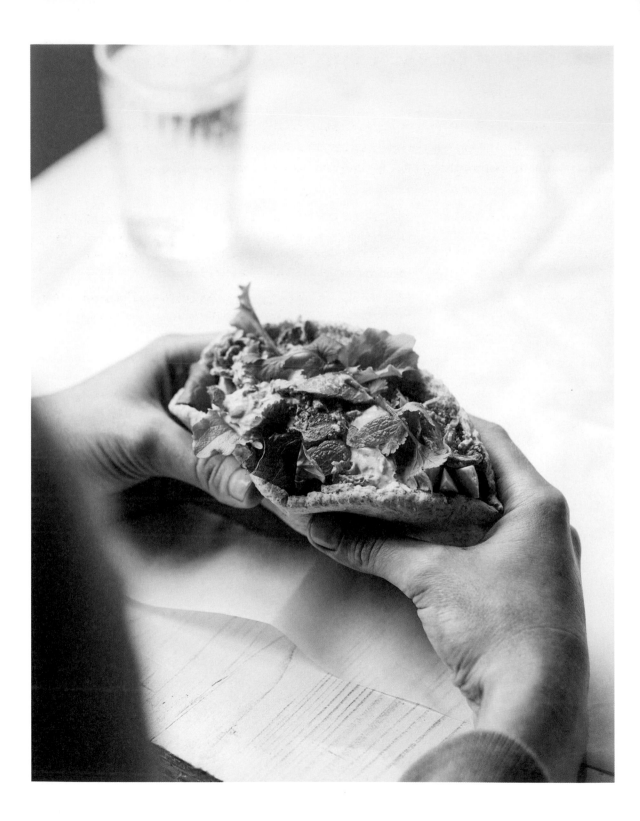

Reinvented saucy mushroom pitta pockets

Plant Points
5.5

Serves **1**   Prep **10 mins**

Pittas are perfect for stuffing in those plant points – literally! These are a great way to have a satisfying and gut-loving lunch on the run using the leftover saucy mushrooms from my filo parcels (page 222), and giving you almost a third of your daily fibre needs.

70g saucy mushroom leftovers, page
    222 (or as much as you can get in)

Toppers:
1 wholemeal pitta (or wrap)
20g salad leaves
50g red pepper, sliced
½ avocado, sliced (approx. 70g)
1 tbsp live thick yoghurt
½ tsp harissa (optional)
fresh herbs (e.g. mint and coriander)

Toast the pitta until warm and slice along a long edge. Stuff with the leaves, red pepper, avocado and the saucy mushrooms. If you prefer your saucy mushrooms warm, heat them in the microwave for a minute or two before adding to your pitta.

Mix the yoghurt with the harissa (if using), then dollop on top of the stuffing with as many fresh herbs as you like.

Switch No peppers to hand? Works well with sliced radish, spring onions or cherry tomatoes.

Storage Best eaten immediately.

Reinvented couscous salad

Serves **2**   Prep **10 mins**

Cook once, eat twice. This simple recipe shows how easy it is to turn leftover roast veg (for example, from the rainbow roast with green Yorkshire puds on page 251) into a whole new meal. The flavoursome combo of spices does all the heavy lifting; you just need to chop, pour and combine . . . and let the flavour take your imagination to sunny Morocco.

200g couscous
1 tsp ras el hanout (or 1 tsp cumin and
   ½ tsp cinnamon)
¼ tsp turmeric
250ml vegetable stock, hot
2 tbsp extra virgin olive oil
10 dried apricots, chopped (approx. 60g)
40g raisins
1 x 400g tin of chickpeas, drained
   and rinsed
15g coriander, chopped
300–400g leftover roast veg, diced
40g almonds, chopped (optional)
100g cherry tomatoes, chopped
   (optional)

Topper:
50g live thick yoghurt (optional)

Place the couscous in a mixing bowl, along with the ras el hanout and turmeric. Pour over the hot stock and olive oil and stir to combine. Cover the bowl with an upturned plate for 5 minutes, and then use a fork to fluff up the grains.

Add all the remaining ingredients to the couscous, season to taste and mix to combine. Top with live thick yoghurt (if using) before tucking in.

Switch Not keen on raisins? Switch for goji berries.

Storage Will keep in the fridge for 2 days.

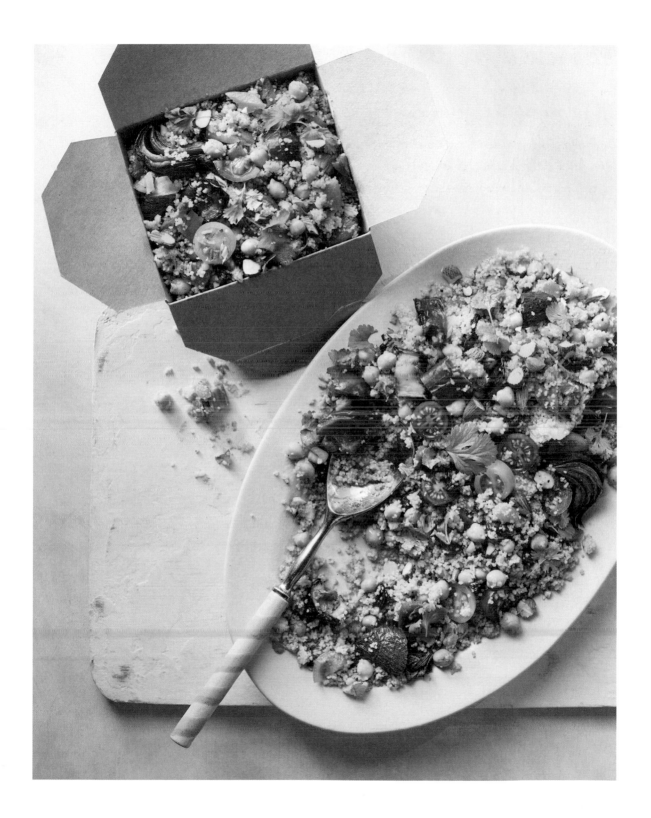

Thai-inspired fishcakes and crunchy salad

Plant Points
6.5

Serves **2**   Prep **10 mins**   Cook **10 mins**

 FODMAP Lite   **Freezer**

Because plant-based doesn't mean *only* plants. This dish celebrates the gut-loving omega-3-filled salmon, and is packed full of plant flavours and colours. You'll want to make a double batch of these to fill your freezer.

Fishcakes:
175g (drained weight) tinned pink or red salmon, or fish of choice
½ tbsp extra virgin olive oil
10g fresh ginger, peeled and roughly chopped
1 stick of fresh lemongrass, roughly chopped (approx. 15g), or 2 tsp lemongrass paste
3 spring onions, roughly chopped (approx. 30g)
½ red chilli, roughly chopped (approx. 20g), or 1 full chilli if you like it spicy (optional)
10g fresh coriander, roughly chopped
10g desiccated coconut
1 large egg
sesame oil, for frying

Salad:
150g bag of salad mix (or 40g watercress, or leaves of choice, 50g grated carrot, 60g shredded cabbage)
5g mixed fresh herbs of choice (coriander, Thai basil, mint)

Dressing:
2g fresh ginger, finely grated
juice of 1 lime (approx. 25 ml)
1 tbsp soy sauce
1 tsp honey
a pinch of dried chilled flakes (optional)

Place all the ingredients for the fishcakes (olive oil, ginger, lemongrass, spring onions, chilli, coriander, coconut and egg) except for the fish and sesame oil in a food processor, and pulse until you have a fairly smooth mix. Scrape down the sides a couple of times to make sure it is all blitzed evenly. Add a pinch of salt and pepper before forking in the fish.

Heat some sesame oil in a frying pan on a low-medium heat. Using wet hands, divide the mix into 4, shape each one into a fishcake and place in the pan. Fry gently for 4–5 minutes each side with the lid on, until cooked through and golden brown.

While the fishcakes are cooking, add the salad ingredients to a large bowl. Mix the dressing ingredients together, before pouring it over the salad.

Serve the fishcakes with the salad and chilli sauce (if using).

Storage   The cooked fishcakes will keep for 3 days in the fridge. Or you can freeze them (cooked) for up to 1 month; defrost and reheat in the microwave or oven. The salad dressing will keep for 1 week in the fridge.

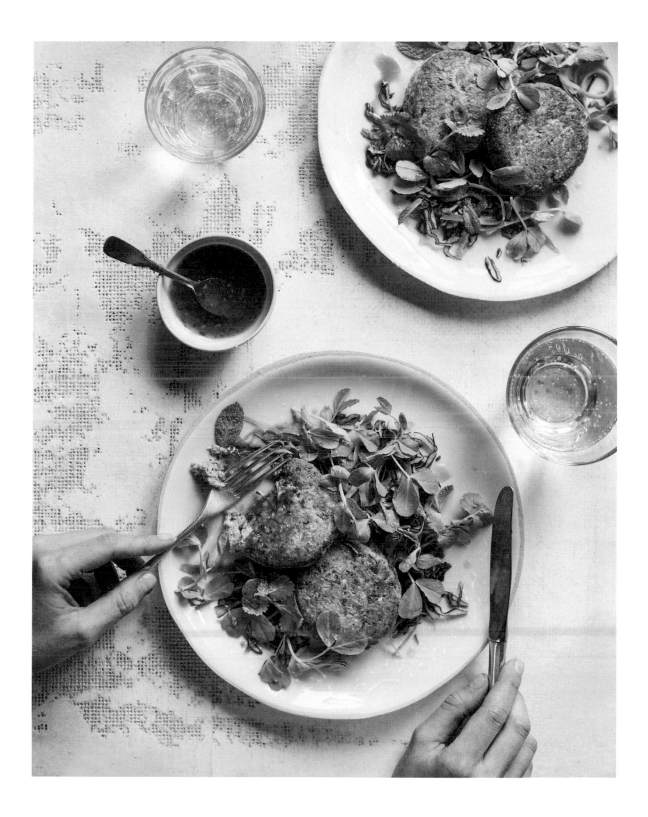

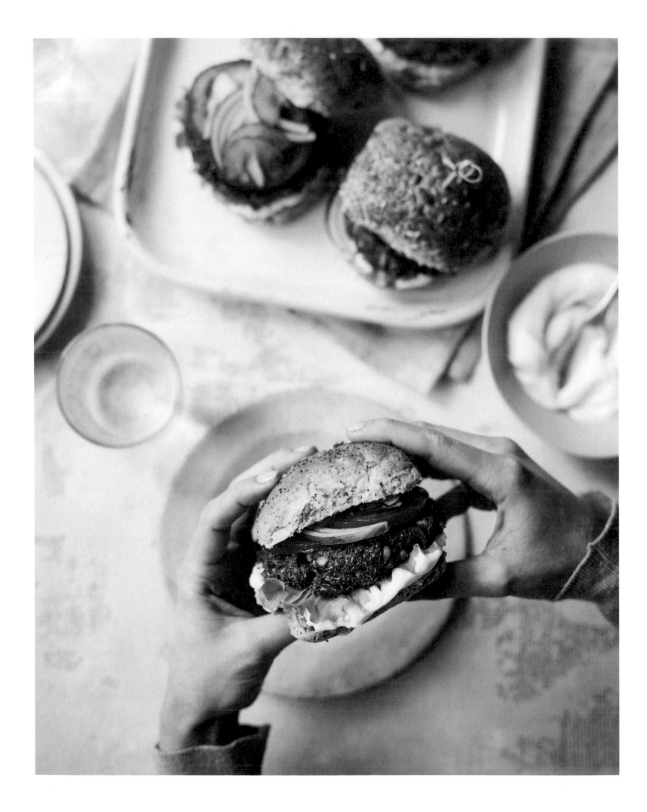

Smoky beet burger

Plant Points
10

Serves **6**   Prep **20 mins**   Cook **10 mins**

 Freezer

I like to think this is a pretty convincing alternative to a beef burger, with a delicious and nutritious twist. The smoky flavour and juicy texture, packed full of 10 plant points, is guaranteed to make this a firm favourite in any meat-loving household. Each burger offers your microbes three times more fibre than your standard burger!

40g ground flaxseed
100g pine nuts, roughly chopped
100g leek, finely chopped
2 garlic cloves, grated or chopped
  (approx. 8g)
2 whole beetroots (approx. 200g)
2 tsp smoked paprika
80g precooked quinoa
6 sundried tomato halves, preserved in
  oil (approx. 50g), finely chopped
90g feta
2 tsp arrowroot (or cornflour)
extra virgin olive oil, for frying

Quick pickles (optional):
1 red onion, sliced (approx. 120g)
½ cucumber, sliced (approx. 120g)
3 tbsp cider vinegar
½ tbsp sea salt
1 tbsp coriander seeds

Toppers:
6 wholegrain seedy buns
garlicky aquafaba aioli (page 170)
3 tomatoes
6 large lettuce leaves

Add all the pickle ingredients to a heatproof bowl (onions, cucumber, vinegar, salt and coriander seeds) with just enough boiling water to cover.

For the burgers, combine the flaxseed with 40ml of boiling water. Set aside to allow it to thicken.

Meanwhile, in a frying pan, toast the pine nuts for 2 minutes. Tip on to a plate and set aside.

Heat some oil in the same frying pan, on a medium heat, and cook the leek and garlic for a few minutes to brown a little.

In a mixing bowl, grate the beetroot. Squeeze out any excess liquid using a strainer.

To the grated beetroot, add all the burger ingredients (fried leek and garlic, pine nuts, paprika, quinoa, flaxseed, sundried tomatoes, feta and arrowroot). Use your hands to mix everything together (a pair of gloves comes in handy here, to stop your hands becoming stained). Taste and season to preference. Using wet, clean hands, divide into six (approx. 100g each) and shape into burgers, squeezing the mixture tightly together as you shape. If still a little too soft, sprinkle in some extra flaxseed.

Add a thin layer of oil to the frying pan, before adding the burgers. Cook for 5 minutes with the lid on, then gently flip the burgers, before cooking for a further 5 minutes.

Once cooked, make the buns up with some aioli, salad, quick pickles and any other favourite toppers.

Storage These can be made ahead of time and refrigerated for up to 3 days. They can also be frozen, raw, for up to 1 month.

Weeknight
Dinners

Stir-fry adventures

Serves **2**   Prep **5 mins**   Cook **5–10 mins**

 FODMAP Lite   **Fridge raid**

Don't underestimate the power of a stir fry when it comes to reaching your plant-point goals during those time-poor weeks – they're a staple on my menu. Although traditionally a Chinese cuisine, using my stir-fry guide you'll see just how easy it is to fuse different flavours from other cultures to create a week's worth of diverse, tasty and quick stir-fry dishes.

Choose one cuisine flavour, one protein, one wholegrain and one vegetable from the list below. Then follow the methods under your cuisine of choice for the ultimate stir-fry adventure.

Cuisine flavour
- Indian
- Italian
- Korean
- Indonesian
- Thai

Protein (approx. 180g)
- tofu
- lentils
- butter beans
- borlotti beans
- cannellini beans

Wholegrain (approx. 200g, cooked)
- mixed wholegrains
- barley
- wheat grains
- rice noodles
- buckwheat noodles
- sourdough bread

Veg (approx. 300g, raw)
- e.g. water chestnuts, bamboo shoots, cabbage, onions, pak choi, bean sprouts, mushrooms, sweetcorn, peppers

Flavour of India

Plant Points **8**

Serves **2**   Prep **5 mins**   Cook **10 mins**

 FODMAP Lite   **Fridge raid**

Cuisine flavour:
8g fresh ginger, grated or crushed
2 garlic cloves, grated or crushed (approx. 8g)
¼ tsp turmeric
1 tsp ground coriander
1 tsp ground cumin
1½ tbsp extra virgin olive oil

Additional veg (optional):
100g cauliflower, roughly chopped

Toppers (optional):
30g almonds, chopped
½ tsp chilli flakes
5g coriander leaves

Add all the cuisine flavour ingredients to a medium frying pan/wok on a medium heat along with the cauliflower (if using). Cook for 3–4 minutes, adding a splash of water if it starts to stick.

Add your stir-fry veg and cook for another 5 minutes until the veg are just cooked, they should still have a little crunch to them. In the final few minutes, stir in your protein and wholegrains of choice. Taste and adjust seasoning.

Serve with your preferred combination of almonds, chilli and coriander leaves.

Tip Pairs well with cooked lentils and your rice of choice.

Storage Keeps in the fridge for up to 3 days.

Flavour of Italy

Plant Points
8

Serves **2**   Prep **5 mins**   Cook **5 mins**

 FODMAP Lite   **Fridge raid**

Cuisine flavour:
3 tbsp extra virgin olive oil
2 garlic cloves, grated
   or crushed
1 tsp small capers, roughly
   chopped
30g Parmesan, grated, or 1½
   tbsp nutritional yeast
   (approx. 7g)
1 tbsp Italian or mixed herbs
juice of ½ lemon (approx. 25ml
   plus zest to taste)

Additional vegetables (optional):
100g cherry tomatoes, halved

Topper:
20g pine nuts

Add all the cuisine flavour ingredients (except for the Parmesan and lemon) to a medium frying pan/wok on a medium heat, along with your stir-fry veg and cook for 5 minutes. In the final 2 minutes, stir in the cherry tomatoes (if using), Parmesan and your protein of choice.

Scatter the pine nuts on top and serve alongside your wholegrain of choice.

Tip Pairs well with Tenderstem broccoli stir-fry mix, cannellini or borlotti beans, and sourdough bread on the side.

Flavour of Korea

Plant Points
7.25

Serves **2**   Prep **5 mins**   Cook **5–10 mins**

 FODMAP Lite   **Fridge raid**

Cuisine flavour:
1½ tbsp sesame oil
1½ tbsp gochujang paste
   or sriracha
1 tbsp soy sauce
1 tbsp mirin (optional)
¼ tsp chilli flakes (optional)

Additional veg (optional):
½ aubergine (approx. 150g),
   sliced into 1cm strips
2 tbsp extra virgin olive oil

Topper (optional):
1 tbsp mixed sesame seeds,
   black or white

Add all the cuisine flavour ingredients to a medium frying pan/wok on a medium heat, along with the aubergine and extra oil (if using) and cook for 5 minutes. If not using the aubergine, add the stir-fry veg straight away.

Add the stir-fry veg mix, and cook for another 5 minutes until the veg are just cooked through, they should have a little crunch to them. In the final few minutes, stir in your chosen protein. Season to taste.

Plate on top of your wholegrains of choice, and finish by sprinkling with the sesame seeds (if using).

Tip Pairs well with tofu and wheat berries or barley.

Storage Keeps in the fridge for up to 3 days.

Flavour of Indonesia

Serves **2**   Prep **10 mins**   Cook **5 mins**

 FODMAP Lite   **Fridge raid**

Cuisine flavour:
2 shallots, finely chopped (approx. 40g)
1 stick lemongrass, roughly chopped, or 1 tsp lemongrass paste
8g fresh ginger, roughly chopped (optional)
½ tsp turmeric (optional)
160ml coconut cream
1 tbsp soy sauce
juice of 1 lime (approx. 25ml)
3 tbsp crunchy peanut butter
sesame oil, for frying

Additional veg (optional):
50g baby corn
50g green beans

Toppers (optional):
1 tbsp roasted peanuts, chopped (approx. 20g)
1 tsp chilli flakes

Place all the cuisine flavour ingredients, except the peanut butter and oil, in a high-powered blender and blitz for 1–2 minutes until smooth. Stir in the peanut butter.

Add the sesame oil to a medium frying pan/wok on a medium heat, along with the stir-fry veg (and additional veg, if using) and mix. Cook for 5 minutes until the veg are just cooked, they should still have a little crunch to them. In the final few minutes, stir in half the cuisine flavour mix from above along with your protein and wholegrains of choice.

Stir through the remaining cuisine flavour mix gradually until you're happy with the consistency and flavour. Scatter the peanuts and chilli flakes on top to serve.

Tip Pairs well with tofu (or cooked chicken or turkey) and buckwheat noodles.

Storage Any leftover satay mix keeps in the fridge for up to 1 week. The stir-fry keeps in the fridge for up to 3 days.

Flavour of Thailand

Serves **2**   Prep **5 mins**   Cook **2–5 mins**

 FODMAP Lite   **Fridge raid**

Cuisine flavour:
8g ginger, peeled and roughly chopped
2 garlic cloves, roughly chopped (approx. 8g)
4 spring onions (approx. 45g)
10g fresh coriander
1 lemongrass stalk, roughly chopped, or 1 tsp lemongrass paste
3 tbsp oyster sauce
1 tbsp fish sauce
1 tbsp olive oil

Additional veg (optional):
100g sugar snap peas or mangetout, left whole

Toppers (optional):
juice of 1 lime (approx. 25ml), or to taste
fresh basil or Thai basil leaves, to taste

Place all the cuisine flavour ingredients except the oil in a high-speed blender and blitz for 1–2 minutes until smooth. Add the oil to a medium frying pan/wok on a medium heat with the sauce and cook for 1 minute.

Add in your stir-fry veg mix (along with additional veg, if using). Cook for 5 minutes until the veg are just cooked, they should still have a little crunch to them. In the final few minutes, stir in your protein and wholegrains of choice. Season to taste.

Top with the lime juice and fresh herbs to taste (if using).

Tip Pairs well with butter beans and rice noodles.

Storage Keeps in the fridge for up to 3 days.

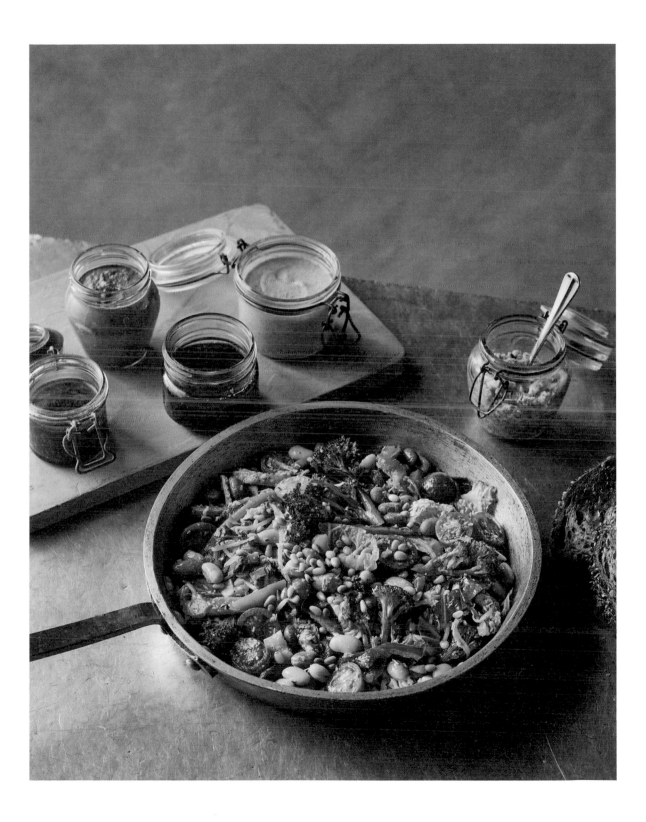

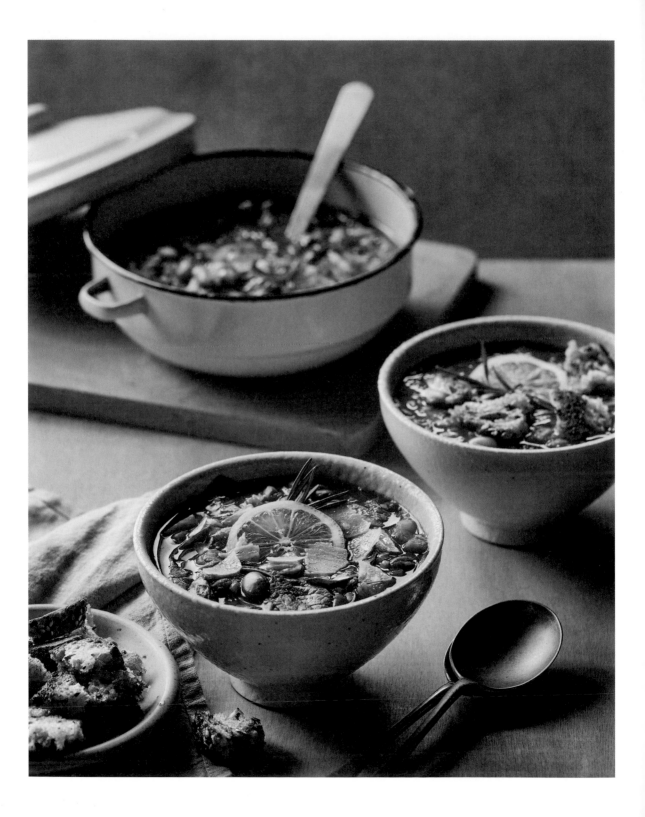

Mediterranean hug soup

Plant Points
10.75

Serves **4**   Prep **10 mins**   Cook **15–30 mins (depending on the type of wholegrain)**

 Freezer

Everything that's great about the Mediterranean captured in a bowl. The heart-warming atmosphere, the flavours, the comfort . . . and, of course, the good gut health. With nearly half your daily fibre needs and a load of prebiotics, your microbes will fall in love with the Med way of life too.

1 tbsp extra virgin olive oil
2 leeks, roughly chopped (approx. 300g)
2 celery sticks, roughly chopped
  (approx. 100g)
1 large carrot, roughly chopped
  (about 120g)
2 garlic cloves, roughly chopped
  (approx. 8g)
1 x 400g tin of chopped tomatoes
1.5 litres vegetable stock
1 fresh sprig rosemary (approx. 9g),
  or ½ tsp of dried rosemary
2 bay leaves
2 x 400g tins of mixed beans, strained
  and rinsed
100g wholegrain of choice, raw, e.g.
  freekeh, or 250g precooked

Toppers (optional):

2 tbsp extra virgin olive oil
100g seeded sourdough bread, or bread
  of choice
50g baby spinach leaves, roughly
  chopped
2 fresh sprigs rosemary, halved (for
  presentation)
Parmesan cheese, grated or shaved
½ lemon, sliced into four circles

Heat the olive oil in a large saucepan and add the leek, celery, carrot and garlic, then cook on a medium-high heat for 5 minutes.

Remove from the heat and add the tinned tomatoes. Using a hand blender, blitz for 30 seconds or until roughly blended (still with some texture). You can do this in the saucepan to save on washing-up.

Next add the vegetable stock, rosemary, bay leaves, mixed beans and wholegrain of choice. Season to taste, then bring up to a gentle boil.

Cook with the lid on until the grains are tender (typically 25 minutes for raw or 10 minutes for precooked/quick-cook grains). Stir occasionally to prevent anything catching on the bottom and add a splash of water if you prefer a thinner soup.

A few minutes before the soup is ready, heat 2 tbsp of olive oil in a frying pan, tear or chop the bread into chunks and add to the pan. Fry until lightly toasted.

Once the soup is ready, remove the bay leaves, stir through the spinach leaves to wilt and season to taste.

Ladle into bowls and top each one with the croutons, rosemary, Parmesan and a slice of lemon (if using).

Switch In the summer months, try swapping the rosemary for some fresh basil or parsley as a lighter alternative.

Storage The soup can be refrigerated for 3 days and frozen for up to 1 month.

Tip Short on time? Try the quick-cook grains now available from most leading supermarkets.

Filo parcels with saucy mushrooms

Serves **2** Makes **9 parcels (with approx. 140g left over to make 2 stuffed pittas the next day)** Prep **15 mins** Cook **15 mins**

The visual appeal of a delicate entrée, but the nourishment and comfort of a main course. These 100 per cent plant-based parcels are sure to be a hit with the whole family. And it gets better – page 207 shows you how to turn the leftover mushroom mix into a tasty lunch.

1 tbsp extra virgin olive oil
½ onion, diced (approx. 75g prepped)
200g mixed mushrooms (e.g. white, portobello, button)
50g cabbage, grated or shredded, or greens of choice
50g carrot, grated
1 garlic clove, grated or crushed (approx. 4g)
1 tbsp harissa
100g silken tofu, roughly chopped
50g walnuts, chopped
75g soy yoghurt, or yoghurt of choice

Pastry parcels:
4 sheets of filo pastry
extra virgin olive oil, for brushing

Preheat the oven to *210°C/190°C fan/gas mark 6* and line a baking tray with non-stick baking paper.

To save on chopping, add the mushrooms to a food processor and roughly pulse to form a chunky mince texture. Heat the oil for the mushroom mix in a large saucepan on a high heat. Cook the onion and the mushrooms for approx. 5 minutes, stirring frequently, until the mushrooms have greatly reduced in volume and the liquid has evaporated.

Add the cabbage, carrot, garlic and harissa, and stir to combine. Cook for a minute or two until the cabbage is just softened, then remove from the heat. Add the tofu, walnuts and yoghurt, and mix to combine. Taste and season to preference. Keep to one side.

Unroll the filo on to a clean worktop and brush 2 sheets all over with olive oil. Add another layer of sheets on top, so you have 2 double sheets. Using the 2 double sheets, create a 45cm x 45cm square, overlapping the 2 double sheets as needed. Be sure to brush the overlapping areas with the oil to help them stick.

Using a sharp knife, cut into 3 columns and 3 rows, making 9 squares. Place a spoonful (approx. 40g of filling) in the middle of each section of pastry, brush around the filling with a little olive oil, then gently pull up the edges to make a parcel. Scrunch into place.

Place them all on a lined baking tray and then bake in the oven for 10 minutes, or until the filo is a deep golden brown.

Storage Best eaten warm out of the oven for the ultimate crispy filo. Keeps in the fridge for up to 3 days. Just reheat in the oven for 5 minutes to get that filo crunch back.

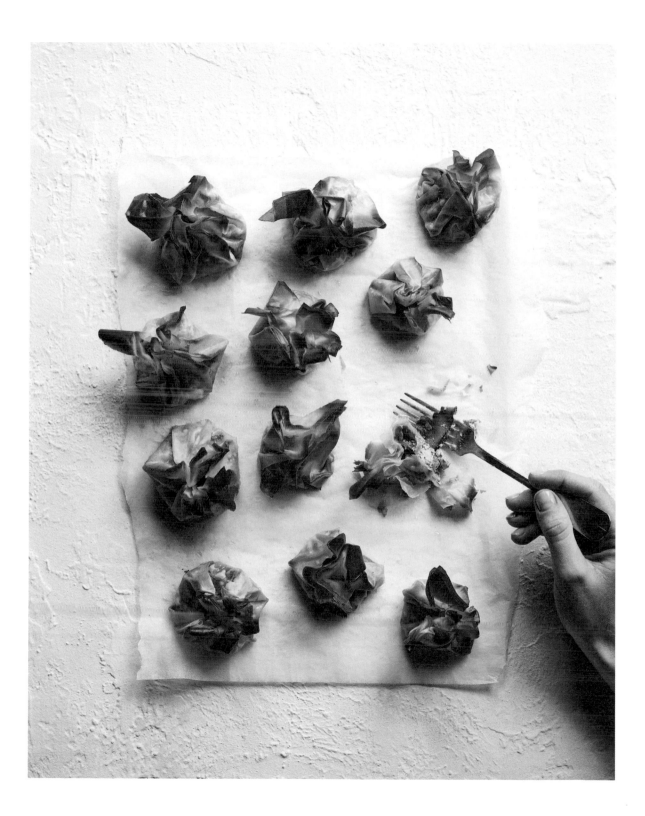

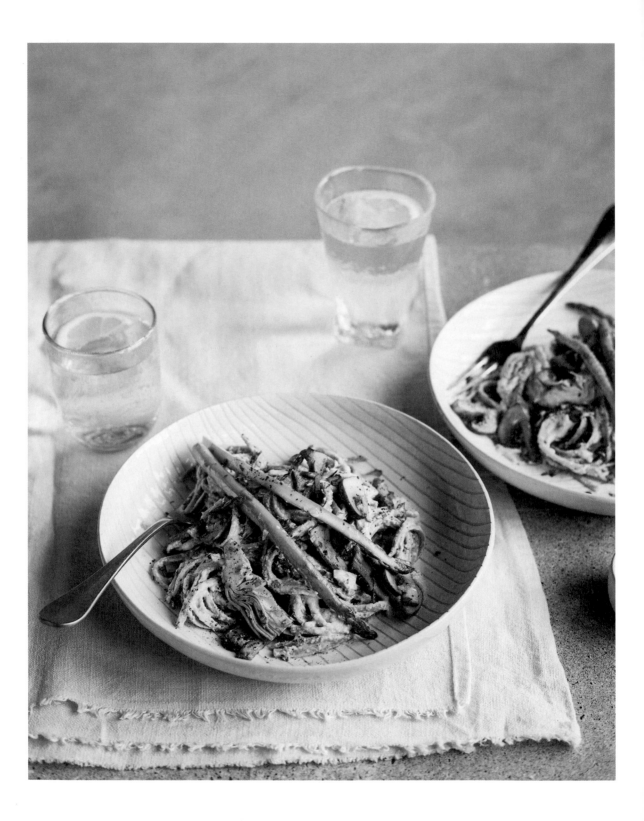

Creamy dairy-free linguine

Plant Points
7.25

Serves **4** Prep **10 mins** Cook **15 mins**

 Zero waste

Turns out it is possible to make a creamy pasta with nothing but plants. The silken tofu and cashew cream pair perfectly with the prebiotic artichokes, mushrooms and asparagus.

240g wholewheat linguine, or pasta of choice

1 shallot or 30g red onion, finely chopped

160g artichoke hearts, preserved in oil

200g chestnut mushrooms, roughly chopped, or mushrooms of choice

150g asparagus spears, cut in half lengthways

Sauce:

100g cashews

250g silken tofu

juice of ½ lemon (approx. 25ml), plus 1 tsp zest

3 tbsp nutritional yeast (approx. 15g)

20g basil leaves, finely chopped

Soak the cashews in 100ml boiling water. Set aside for at least 10 minutes.

Bring a large saucepan of water to the boil and add a big pinch of salt. Add the pasta and cook for 10 minutes (or according to packet instructions).

While the pasta is boiling, heat 2 tbsp of the oil from the artichoke hearts in a large frying pan and add the shallots. Cook for 2 minutes before adding the artichoke hearts, mushrooms and asparagus. Cook over a medium-high heat for 5 minutes, or until the mushrooms have started to become golden brown and the asparagus is al dente. If you want to impress on presentation, set aside a third of this veg mix to add on top of the plated dish.

Place all the ingredients for the sauce (except the basil) in a high-powered food processor, including the water the cashews have been soaking in. Blitz for 5 minutes until smooth, scraping the sides down occasionally. Stir in the basil, add extra zest and season to taste.

Drain the pasta (reserving a couple of spoonfuls of the pasta water), and add to the veg in the frying pan along with the creamy sauce. Toss to combine, adding a splash of the reserved pasta water to thin the sauce if you need to.

Heat through for a minute or so before dividing between your serving dishes, and finish with a grind of black pepper and any reserved veg mix.

Tip Using the oil that veg are preserved in (like the artichoke hearts) can add a real kick of flavour, as the veg have marinated and flavoured it – plus there's zero waste!

Switch After an extra plant point? Add 50g of pine nuts in the final 2 minutes of the veg cooking.

Storage The sauce keeps in the fridge for up to 1 week. The whole dish keeps for up to 3 days in the fridge.

Orange-glazed roasted salmon

Plant Points **13.25**

Serves **4**   Prep **10 mins**   Cook **20 mins**

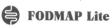 **FODMAP Lite**

A celebration of omega-3 – one nutrient many of us overlook for gut health. This roasted salmon with orange glaze is the perfect reminder that health and flavour absolutely can go hand in hand. If you have the extra time, it's best served with a side of sticky parsnips (page 264) along with the wholegrains and greens.

4 x salmon fillets, skin on (approx.
   130–150g each)
1 tbsp toasted sesame oil
½ tbsp soy sauce
400g greens of choice (e.g. pak choi,
   spring greens or sliced kale)
500g precooked mixed wholegrains, or
   wholegrains of choice
2 spring onions, sliced
1 red chilli, deseeded and finely sliced
   (optional)

Marinade (triple this if making the parsnips):
juice of ½ orange (approx. 40ml)
1 garlic clove, grated
10g ginger, grated
1½ tbsp soy sauce
½ tbsp sesame oil
1 Medjool date, mixed to a paste (see
   page 134), or 1 tbsp sweetener of
   choice

To serve:
1 tbsp sesame seeds
sticky parsnips (page 264) (optional)

Preheat the oven to *220°C/200°C fan/gas mark 7*.

Place all the ingredients for the marinade in a small saucepan, bring to the boil for 5 minutes, stirring frequently, until reduced and syrupy.

Meanwhile, with foil make four little 'bowls' for the salmon to go in, and place on a baking tray. Add one piece of salmon to each foil 'bowl' and, when ready, coat with the reduced marinade, before folding up the foil.

Place in the oven and bake for 10 minutes, opening the foil for the final 5 minutes to brown a little. Check the fish is cooked (the flesh should be opaque all the way through; if it still looks translucent, return to the oven for 2 more minutes).

While the fish is in the oven, heat the sesame oil and the soy sauce in a frying pan over a medium heat before adding your greens of choice. Cook until softened (approx. 5 minutes).

Add the cooked wholegrains, spring onion and sliced chilli (if using) to the pan and cook for a couple of minutes to heat through.

Divide the wholegrains between your serving plates, along with the sticky parsnips (if using), and top with the greens, salmon and any juices from the foil bowls. Sprinkle with sesame seeds.

Tip After crispy salmon skin? Finish the salmon off in the frying pan, skin-side down, over a medium heat for the last 5 minutes.

Storage Keeps in the fridge for up to 3 days.

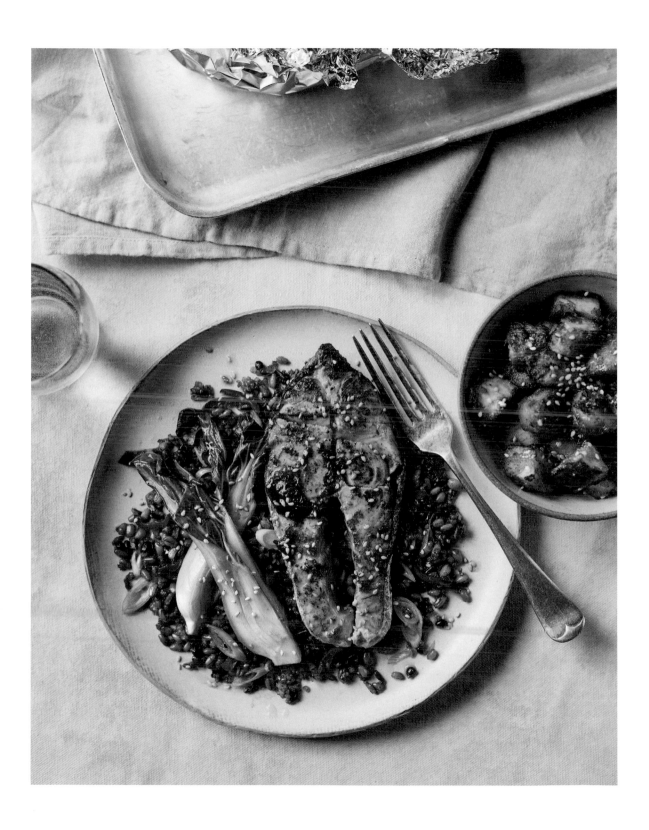

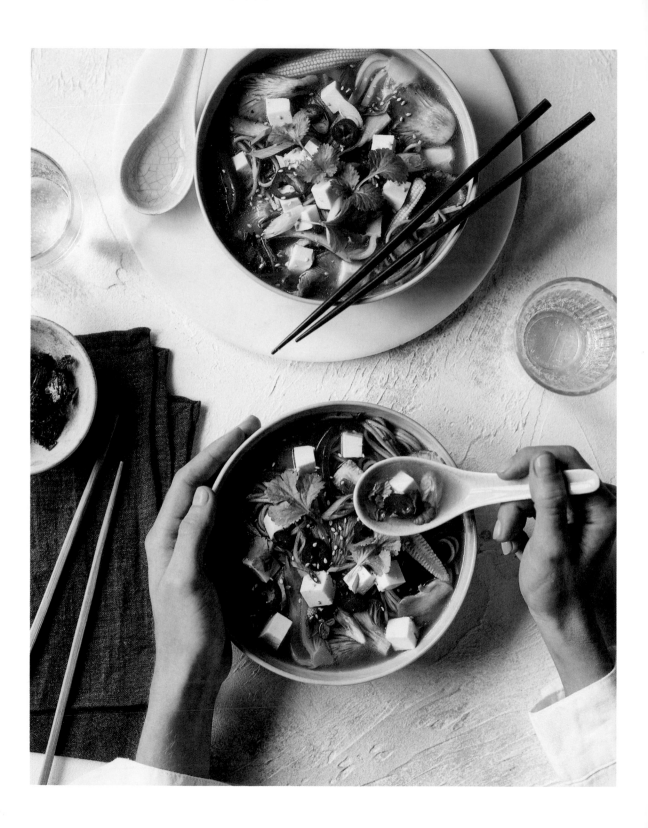

Easy noodle broth

Plant Points
9

Serves **2**   Prep **10 mins**   Cook **10 mins**

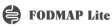 **FODMAP Lite**

Craving a pot of noodles? Let me tempt you with this flavourful alternative that will leave you and your microbes feeling warm and fuzzy inside. It's also a great way to use up any leftover bits of veg, as the broth will give them a new lease of life.

1 litre vegetable stock

1 tbsp soy sauce

15g ginger

2 whole star anise

10g fresh coriander

150g dried soba noodles or 300g non-dried noodles, or noodles of choice

150g pak choi, halved lengthways

1 tbsp sesame oil

8 baby corn, halved longthways (approx. 100g)

½ red pepper, sliced (approx. 80g)

150g oyster mushrooms

200g silken tofu, cut into bite-size cubes

To serve:

1 red chilli, finely sliced (approx. 15g), to taste

1 spring onion, finely sliced (approx. 15g)

½ tbsp sesame seeds

½ tsp nori seaweed flakes (optional)

Place the stock in a large saucepan and place on a medium heat, adding in the soy sauce, knob of ginger and star anise.

Finely chop the coriander stalks and add these to the stock, saving the leaves for a garnish. Bring the stock to the boil and simmer for 5 minutes, then add the soba noodles and cook to packet instructions (usually around 5 minutes). Add the pak choi for the final 2 minutes.

While the noodles are cooking in the broth, heat the sesame oil in a frying pan and, when hot, add the corn, red pepper and mushrooms. Toss around the pan to make sure they cook evenly for approx. 5 minutes.

Divide the noodles and pak choi between two bowls and pour the broth over the top (discarding the ginger and star anise). Then add the tofu (it will warm through in the broth) and divide the veg between the two bowls.

Sprinkle with the chilli, spring onion, sesame seeds and nori flakes (if using), and finally add the reserved coriander leaves.

Storage Best eaten immediately, but can be kept in the fridge for 2 days.

Super green pea and 'ham' soup

Plant Points
11.25

Serves **4**   Prep **10 mins**   Cook **10 mins**

 Freezer

A plant-based play on pea and ham soup. This colour-popping creamy pea soup delivers around half your daily fibre needs per portion. The crispy coconut 'ham', hint of mint and sweetness from the peas takes things to the next level. And the appeal doesn't stop there – it's also perfect for warming your hands around on a winter's day.

1 tbsp extra virgin olive oil
1 onion, chopped (approx. 180g)
3 sticks celery, chopped (approx. 110g)
3 garlic cloves, sliced (approx. 12g)
400g peas, frozen
150g baby spinach leaves
1 x 400g tin of haricot beans or other white beans, drained
5g mint leaves, or more to taste
850ml vegetable stock, hot

Coconut 'ham':
30g coconut flakes
1 tsp extra virgin olive oil
½ tsp smoked paprika
¼ tsp garlic powder

To serve (optional):
100g live thick yoghurt
4 slices of wheaten bread (page 176), or crusty bread of choice

Preheat the oven to *200°C/180°C fan/gas mark 6* and line a small oven tray with non-stick baking paper.

Heat 1 tbsp of olive oil in a large saucepan and add the onion, celery and garlic. Cook on a low-medium heat for 5 or so minutes until softening but not browning. This helps to bring out the natural sweetness of the veg.

While the veg are sweating, place the coconut flakes, 1 tsp of olive oil, paprika, garlic powder and a pinch of salt into the lined baking tray and toss until all the coconut is coated. Place the tray in the oven for 3–4 minutes until the coconut is golden brown.

Once the onion and celery have softened, add the peas, spinach, beans, mint leaves and hot stock, and stir to combine everything. Bring to the boil and simmer for a few minutes.

Remove the saucepan from the heat and blitz with a hand blender until it reaches your preferred consistency. Season to taste.

Divide the soup into portions and top with the yoghurt (if using) – use a knife to make yoghurt swirls – and some of the coconut 'ham' and crusty bread.

Storage   The soup can be kept in the fridge for up to 3 days, or frozen for up to 1 month.

Tip   For extra-smooth soup, blitz in a high-powered blender for 1–2 minutes before adding the yoghurt and serving.

Loaded vegan nachos

Serves **4**   Prep **10–20 mins + soaking time (depending on optional cashew cheese and toppers)**
Cook **15 mins**

There are few things more satisfying than a tray of loaded nachos with all the trimmings. This is one of my favourites for a fun Friday night. The moreish cheese, guacamole and meaty jackfruit combo makes it hard to stop – but you are eating for trillions of microbes after all.

4 wholemeal pittas (approx. 15cm long)
2 tbsp extra virgin olive oil

Pulled jackfruit:
1 tsp ground cumin
1 tsp garlic powder
1 tsp smoked paprika
1 tbsp soy sauce
¼ tsp ground black pepper
2 tbsp extra virgin olive oil
1 tbsp honey
½ tsp Worcestershire sauce
a pinch of cayenne pepper (optional)
1 x 400g tin of jackfruit, drained
1 x 400g tin of black beans, drained and
   rinsed

Guacamole:
1 avocado (approx. 200g whole)
juice from 1 lime (approx. 25ml)
5g fresh coriander, finely chopped
1 tsp extra virgin olive oil (optional)

Cashew cheese (optional):
150g cashews, soaked in 300ml boiling
   water for at least 30 minutes
3 tbsp nutritional yeast
2 tsp lemon juice
1 tsp Dijon mustard
½ tsp garlic powder
¼ tsp smoked paprika
¼ tsp turmeric

Toppers (optional):
¼ cup aioli from page 170, or yoghurt
1 jalapeño pepper, sliced (approx. 30g)
half a bunch of coriander, roughly
   chopped (approx. 15g)
100g cherry tomatoes, halved
2 limes, cut into wedges

Preheat the oven to *200°C/180°C fan/gas mark 6*, and line a large oven tray with non-stick baking paper.

Cut the pittas in half so you have the two ovals, and then cut into 'tortilla' chips. Drizzle with the olive oil and season with salt. Place on the baking tray and pop in the oven for 10 minutes or until crisp.

While the chips are baking, make the pulled jackfruit. In a small bowl, mix together everything except the jackfruit and black beans (the spices, seasoning, olive oil and honey). Shred the jackfruit with your hands, before coating with the mixture. Set aside to marinate.

To make the guacamole, cut the avocado in half and remove the stone. Spoon the flesh into a small bowl and press with a fork until coarsely mashed. Mix in the lime juice, coriander and olive oil, and season to taste. Leave to one side.

If making, place all the ingredients for the cashew cheese (including the soaking water) in a high-powered blender. Blitz for 3–4 minutes, scraping the sides down occasionally.

To a frying pan on a medium heat, add the marinated jackfruit and cook for 3–5 minutes until slightly charred, adding a splash of water if the jackfruit becomes too dry. Add the black beans for the last minute, before taking off the heat.

Take the baking tray out of the oven and top the warm tortilla chips with the pulled jackfruit, cashew cheese and guacamole, along with whatever other toppers you're going for – yoghurt, fresh herbs, jalapeño slices, tomatoes etc. Serve any remaining cheese in a dish on the side.

Storage   The pulled jackfruit keeps in the fridge for up to 3 days, and cashew cheese keeps well in a sealed container in the fridge for up to 5 days, but the loaded nachos are best eaten straight away.

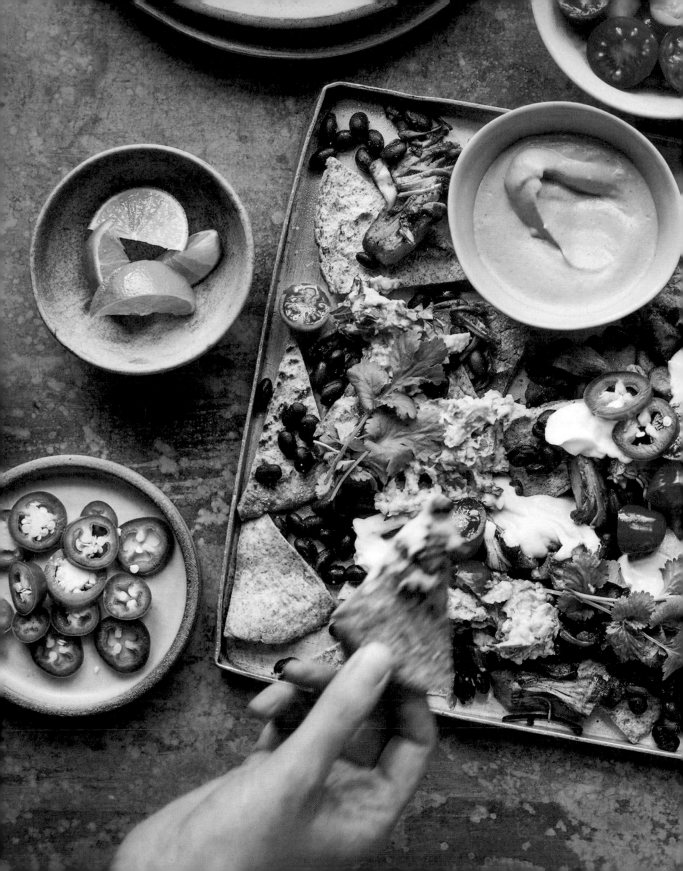

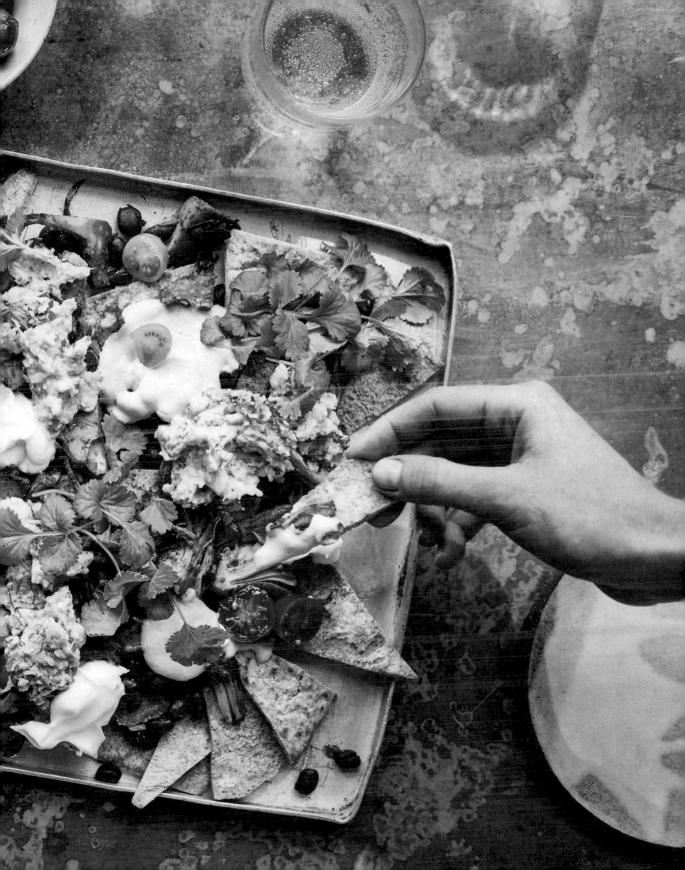

Fancy
Dinners

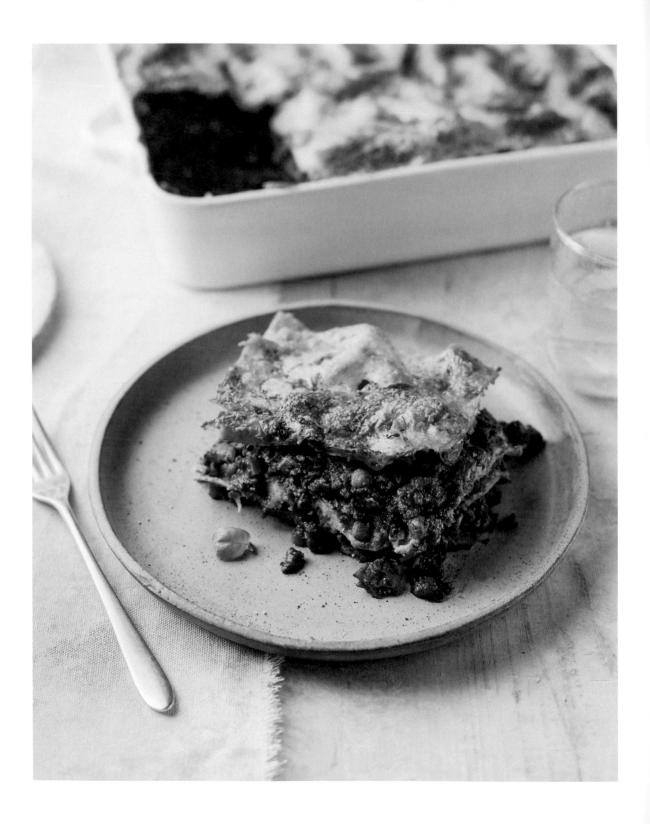

Hearty lasagne

Plant Points
9.25

Serves **8**   Prep **20 mins**   Cook **1 hour**

 Fridge raid   ✳ **Freezer**

The ideal dish to show meat lovers that eating more plants doesn't mean missing out. A comforting family staple that ticks all the flavour boxes with half (or none) of the meat. The versatile ragu can be frozen and used as the base for cottage pie or simply poured over pasta – this is so much more than your average lasagne!

Ragu:
2 tbsp extra virgin olive oil
1 onion, chopped (approx. 180g)
2 carrots, diced (approx. 200g)
2 celery sticks, diced
4 garlic cloves, grated or minced
400g chestnut mushrooms, or mushrooms of choice
300g minced beef (optional)
2 tbsp tomato puree
1 x 400g tin of green lentils, drained and rinsed (or 2 if not using beef)
2 x 400g tins of chopped tomatoes
1 tbsp balsamic vinegar
10g fresh basil, finely chopped
1 tbsp dried mixed herbs
½ tsp ground nutmeg

White sauce:
2 tbsp extra virgin olive oil
45g white flour, or flour of choice
700ml soy milk, or milk of choice
30g grated Parmesan, or cheese of choice
1 tsp Dijon mustard

Layers:
500g dried wholemeal pasta sheets, or pasta sheets of choice
40g baby spinach leaves
40g grated Cheddar, or cheese of choice
5g fresh basil

To make the ragu, heat the olive oil in a large saucepan over a medium heat. Add the onion, carrot, celery and garlic, and cook for 5 minutes until softened and starting to brown. This helps to release the natural sweetness of the veg and develops flavour.

While the veg are cooking, pulse the mushrooms in a food processor until finely chopped, and put to one side.

If you are using meat, add it to the saucepan of veg along with the tomato puree and cook until browned, approx. 5 minutes. Finally, add the remaining ingredients (mushrooms, lentils, chopped tomatoes, balsamic vinegar, basil, mixed herbs and nutmeg).

Stir well and bring up to the boil, before reducing the heat so it gently simmers with the lid on for 15 minutes. Stir occasionally to stop anything catching on the bottom of the pan. You want to end up with a rich sauce, although still with plenty of juice, as this will be soaked up by the pasta sheets. Season to taste.

While the ragu is cooking, make the white sauce by heating the olive oil in a saucepan with the flour. Stir continuously until a paste forms – this is called a roux (this should take approx. 2 minutes). Then slowly start to whisk in the milk in gradual additions. Once all the milk has been added, bring to the boil and simmer for 5 minutes until thickened. Remove from the heat and whisk in the mustard and Parmesan, and season to taste.

When you are ready to start assembling the lasagne, preheat the oven to *180°C/160°C fan/gas mark 4* and lightly oil an ovenproof dish (approx. 28cm x 18cm in size). ➡

Spread a layer of the ragu sauce over the bottom of the dish (approx. one-third), then a layer of lasagne sheets (snapping the sheets if needed, to make them fit), followed by a layer of the white sauce and topped with 20g of the spinach leaves. Repeat these layers 2 more times, but instead of a third layer of spinach leaves, sprinkle the Cheddar over the final layer of white sauce.

Cover with foil and bake in the oven for 30 minutes, removing the foil in the final 10 minutes to crisp up the top. Garnish with the basil leaves before serving.

Aubergine layers

Already had pasta this week? Try switching the pasta sheets for aubergine layers.

3 medium aubergines (approx. 750g)
2 tbsp extra virgin olive oil

To prepare the aubergine layers, preheat the oven to *220°C/200°C fan/ gas mark 7* and line two large baking trays with non-stick baking paper.

While the ragu is cooking, thinly slice the aubergine into 3mm thick slices (use a mandolin if you have one). Lay as many as you can in a single layer on the trays. Brush lightly with olive oil, season, and bake for 8–10 minutes until softened and browning in patches. Repeat with the remaining aubergine slices.

Cook off a little extra of the ragu juice as the aubergine doesn't absorb as much as the pasta sheets. Then lay down the cooked aubergine layers in place of the pasta sheets as described above.

Tip You can serve the ragu by itself over pasta, or use it in a cottage pie – just add 2 tbsp of Worcestershire sauce instead of the balsamic vinegar and leave out the fresh basil.

Storage This will keep for 3 days in the fridge or 2 months in the freezer uncooked; defrost fully in the fridge overnight and bake as per recipe.

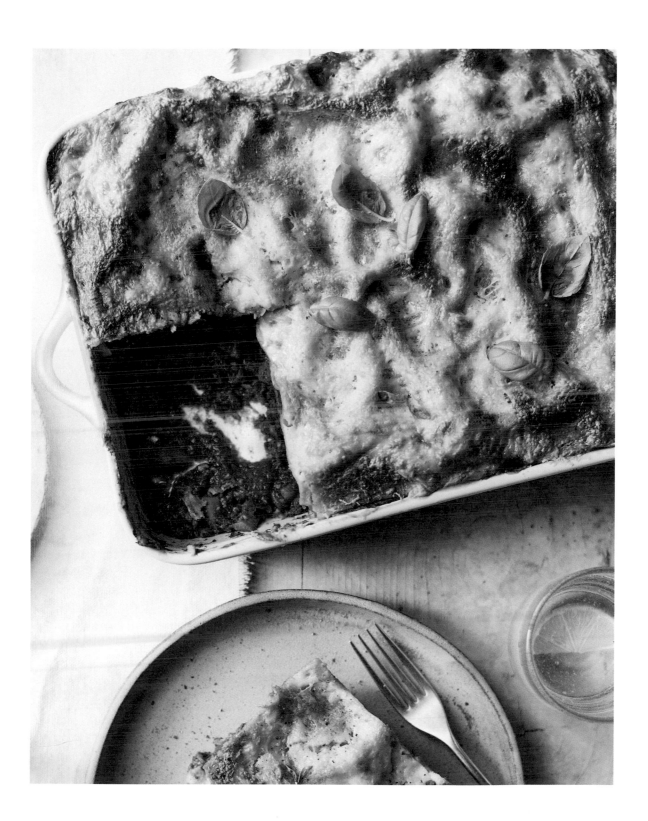

Spicy red lentil bowl

Plant Points
10

Serves **4**   Prep **15 mins**   Cook **25 mins**

 Freezer

This recipe was inspired by my love of dhal and has evolved over the years into this delicious dish with added texture and flavour from the roasted toppings. Serving up to **40 per cent of your daily fibre needs**, this is one tasty way to thriving gut microbes.

2 tbsp extra virgin olive oil
3 garlic cloves, grated
10g ginger, grated
1 green chilli, chopped
1 tsp turmeric
1 tsp ground cumin
8 curry leaves
120g white cabbage, shredded
250g split red lentils, raw
400ml coconut milk
400ml vegetable stock
1 x 400g tin of chopped tomatoes
40g spinach, roughly chopped (optional)

Roasted veg:
2 sweet potatoes (approx. 340g)
2 red onions, cut into 8 wedges
    (approx. 250g)
1 x 400g tin of chickpeas, drained and
    rinsed, or legume of choice
2 tbsp extra virgin olive oil
2 tsp curry powder

Toppers (optional):
a small bunch of coriander, roughly
    chopped (approx. 15g)
30g coconut flakes, toasted
¼ cup live thick yoghurt

Preheat the oven to *220°C/200°C fan/gas mark 7*.

Place the sweet potato in a microwave-safe dish with a splash of water, and cook on high for 5 minutes to soften.

Meanwhile, heat 2 tbsp of oil in a large saucepan and add the garlic, ginger, chilli, turmeric, cumin and curry leaves. Cook for 2–3 minutes until aromatic. If the spices stick, add 1–2 tbsp of water.

Add the cabbage and lentils and stir well to coat them in the spices, before mixing in the coconut milk, stock and chopped tomatoes. Bring up to a gentle boil.

Reduce the heat, then cook with the lid on for 20 minutes or until the lentils are tender. In the final minute, stir in the spinach (if using). Taste and adjust seasoning to preference. Add extra vegetable stock if a little thick.

While the lentils are cooking, transfer the softened sweet potato, as well as the red onion and chickpeas, to a lined tray and drizzle with 2 tbsp of olive oil. Sprinkle with curry powder and season to taste. Toss to combine, before placing in the oven for 20 minutes or until golden brown.

Serve topped with the roasted veg and toppers (if using).

Tip No toasted coconut to hand? All it takes is 1–2 minutes over moderate heat in the frying pan. Be sure to stir the flakes every few seconds to ensure even toasting.

Switch Had enough sweet potato this week? Switch out for aubergine or courgette (no need to microwave the courgette).

Storage Will keep in the fridge for up to 3 days, or in the freezer for 1 month.

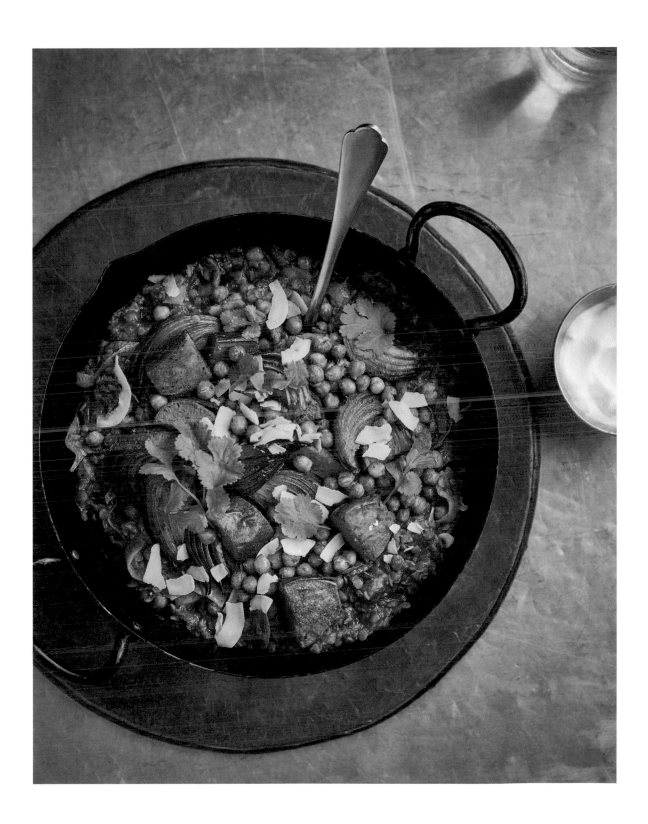

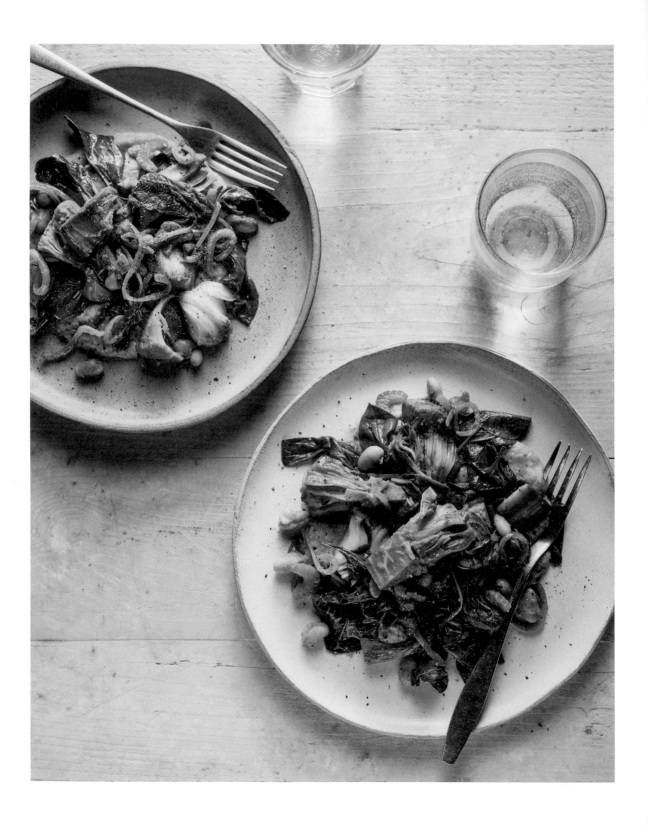

Creamy beans with 'meaty' jackfruit

Serves **2**   Prep **10 mins**   Cook **15 mins**

Forget those processed mock meats and say hello to naturally 'meaty' jackfruit. This hearty (and gut-loving) dish has a prebiotic punch from the bean base, and will give your classic sausage casserole a run for its money.

1 x 560g tin of jackfruit, drained, rinsed and patted dry (dry weight 280g)
1 tbsp extra virgin olive oil
1 small white onion, sliced (approx. 150g)
2 celery sticks, sliced (approx. 80g)
2 garlic cloves, grated (approx. 8g)
250ml vegetable stock
1 x 400g tin of cannellini beans, drained and rinsed
20g Parmesan, grated
60g spinach, or spring greens

Marinade:
1 tbsp Worcestershire sauce
1 tsp marmite
2 tbsp extra virgin olive oil
½ tsp dried rosemary
¼ tsp onion granules

Combine the marinade ingredients in a bowl, before stirring in and coating the jackfruit. Leave to marinate for a few minutes.

Heat the olive oil in a frying pan on a medium heat. Add the onion, celery and garlic, and cook for 5 minutes until everything has started to soften and go golden brown. Transfer half of the onion mix to a high-powered blender, along with the vegetable stock and half of the beans, then blend until smooth. Set aside the other half of the beans and onion mix. Return the blended mix to the frying pan, along with the rest of the stock and the Parmesan, and simmer for 10–15 minutes with the lid off until the stock has reduced. Season to taste. This will be the creamy base of your dish.

While the pureed bean mix is simmering, heat a small frying pan over a medium heat. Tip in the jackfruit with its marinade. Cook for 5–10 minutes, stirring frequently, until the marinade has reduced and the jackfruit is browned. In the final few minutes, add the reserved (non-pureed) onion mix and beans to the frying pan. Stir-fry for a few minutes before adding the greens. Once they have wilted (approx. 1–2 minutes), you're ready to serve.

To each serving bowl, add half the pureed bean mix, topped with the jackfruit stir-fry mix and a grind of black pepper.

Switch No jackfruit? Switch for 300g of mushrooms.

Storage Will keep for 3 days in the fridge.

Sweet potato gnocchi with super pesto

Plant Points
6.75

Serves **4–6 (makes approx. 60 pieces)** Prep **30 mins** Cook **20 mins**

 Freezer

Feeling a little adventurous, but not ready to make pasta from scratch? Foolproof for the novice cook, it's a great way to build your pasta-making confidence. Pan-frying makes them deliciously crispy, but you can enjoy straight from the boiling water with the pesto too.

Gnocchi:
650g sweet potato
350g floury potatoes (e.g. Maris Piper)
150g spelt flour, plus extra to dust
1 tsp turmeric
1 large egg, beaten
200g cherry tomatoes
1 tbsp extra virgin olive oil, plus extra for frying

Pesto:
50g Brussels sprouts
40g fresh basil
50g walnuts
2 tbsp fresh lemon juice, to taste
120ml extra virgin olive oil
50g Parmesan, finely grated

Toppers (optional):
shaved Parmesan

Pierce the sweet and floury potatoes with a fork and cook in the microwave on high for 8–10 minutes until cooked through and soft.

While the potatoes are cooking, start making the pesto. First cook the Brussels sprouts in simmering water for 3 minutes or until just tender. Drain and run under cold water to cool. Place all the ingredients (except for the Parmesan and olive oil) in a food processor, and blitz into a rough paste. Add the lemon juice, oil and Parmesan gradually, one at a time, until you're happy with the consistency and flavour. Season to taste.

Once cool enough to handle, scrape out the insides of the cooked potatoes into a large mixing bowl and either mash or use a potato ricer. Add the flour, turmeric and egg and gently mix together with a butter knife, using a cutting action. This will help prevent the dough getting tough.

Once combined, divide into 4 and roll each into 1.5cm-thick sausages on a lightly floured surface. If too wet to roll, add a little extra flour. Cut the rolls into bite-sized gnocchi.

When you're ready to eat, bring a large saucepan of salted water to the boil and carefully drop in a third of the gnocchi. Once cooked, they'll float to the surface (approx. 2 minutes). Repeat with the remaining gnocchi.

Heat some olive oil in a large frying pan and add the cooked gnocchi to the pan, along with the cherry tomatoes. Toss to coat the gnocchi and cook for a few minutes until they start to brown slightly.

Serve topped with a little more grated Parmesan and a twist of black pepper.

Storage Leftover pesto can be kept in the fridge for up to 1 week if you cover with olive oil or cling film, or frozen for up to 3 months. Fresh gnocchi can be kept in the fridge for up to 2 days, or frozen for 1 month.

Switch Stir pesto into wild rice, wholemeal pasta or shop-bought gnocchi.

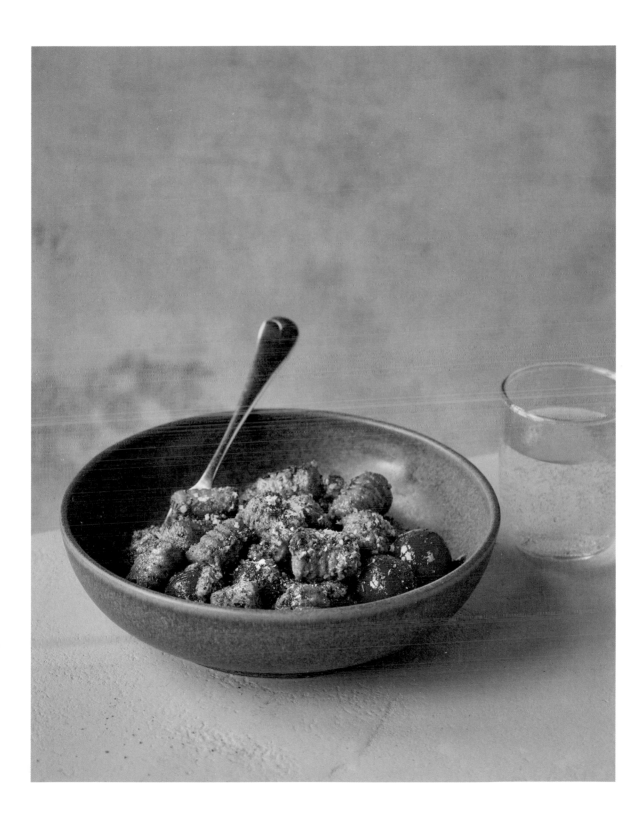

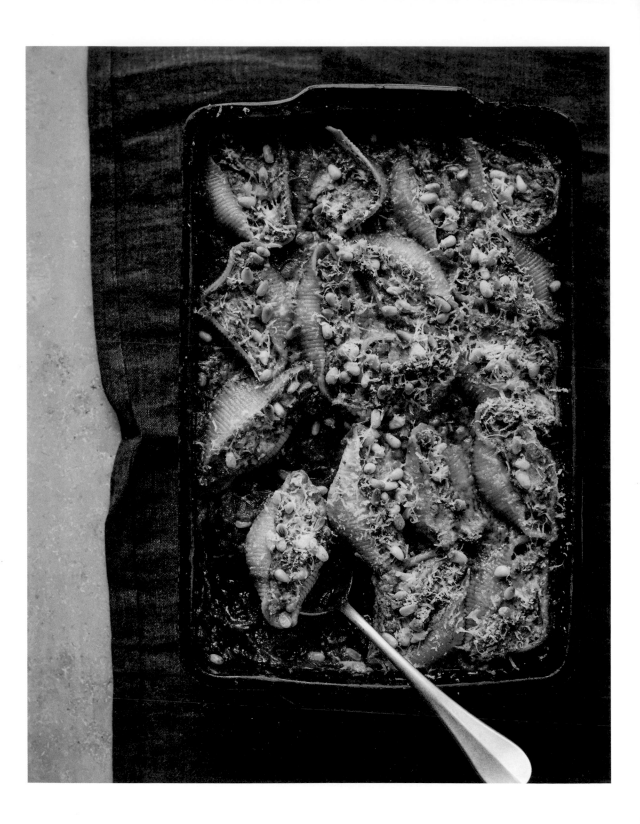

Spinach and ricotta stuffed pasta shells

Plant Points
7.75

Serves **4** Prep **15 mins** Cook **30 mins**

 FODMAP Lite   **Freezer**

Coming from an Italian family, homemade ravioli has always been part of our celebrations. But after moving to London and realizing I didn't have the time or skill, it was either forgo one of my favourites or conjure up an easier and quicker alternative . . . and so these delicious stuffed pasta shells were born. I couldn't let my microbes miss out on the feast, so I've ensured they contain over a third of your daily fibre needs and prebiotics too.

Rich tomato sauce:
1 tbsp extra virgin olive oil
2 garlic cloves, grated
10 sundried tomato halves, preserved in oil, chopped (approx. 85g)
1 x 400g tin of chopped tomatoes
20g basil, roughly chopped
200g passata

Stuffed pasta:
250g fresh spinach
24 conchiglie shells or 12 cannelloni tubes (about 175g)
1 x 400g tin of mixed beans, drained and rinsed
120g peas, fresh or frozen
250g ricotta
150g feta, crumbled

Toppers:
20g pine nuts
20g Parmesan, grated

Heat the olive oil in a saucepan and add the garlic. Cook for a couple of minutes until aromatic and then add the sundried tomatoes, chopped tomatoes, 100ml water, basil, passata and season to taste. Cook on a low heat for around 15 minutes with the lid off.

In the meantime, make the pasta filling by heating a large saucepan and adding the spinach with a splash of water. Place a lid on and let the spinach wilt for a couple of minutes. Then transfer to a sieve and squeeze out the excess water before placing in a food processor. Add the beans and peas, and blitz until roughly smooth (approx. 2 minutes). Stir in the ricotta and feta.

Preheat the oven to *200°C/180°C fan/gas mark 6*.

Lightly oil an ovenproof dish (approx. 25cm x 30cm). Pour in the cooked rich tomato sauce and spread out in an even layer.

Rinse the saucepan and fill with water. Bring to the boil and cook the pasta shells for 2 minutes less than the pack instructions, so they're just cooked and holding their shape. Drain the shells and, once they're cool enough to handle, stuff them with the filling and place all the filled shells in the tomato sauce.

Scatter the pine nuts and grated Parmesan over the top and bake for approx. 20 minutes until golden brown.

Tip Short on time? Scrap the tomato sauce recipe and use your favourite ready-made tomato and basil pasta sauce.

Storage Keeps in the fridge for 3 days. The uncooked filling can keep in the freezer for up to 1 month. Defrost overnight in the fridge, then stuff your shells and cook following the recipe instructions.

Tear-and-share with butter bean relish

Plant Points
6

Serves **4**   Prep **10 mins**   Cook **20 mins**

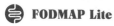 **FODMAP Lite**

A favourite dinner party dish that everyone can tuck into. The crispy sea-salted bread encasing a sticky, plant-filled relish served straight out of the oven will be the talk of the table. It's the perfect opening to introduce your guests to their inner universe of microbes, if they're still outsiders.

Filling:

2 tbsp extra virgin olive oil
1 large onion, finely chopped
1 sprig rosemary, leaves picked and
   finely chopped
1 tbsp balsamic vinegar
½ tbsp Worcestershire sauce
2 Medjool dates, made into a paste
   (see page 134), or 2 tbsp sweetener
1 x 400g tin of chopped tomatoes
1 tsp wholegrain mustard
½ tsp smoked paprika
1 x 400g tin of butter beans, drained
   and rinsed
20g Parmesan (optional), plus extra
   for topping

To serve:

1 cob loaf (approx. 400g)
extra virgin olive oil, for drizzling
   and brushing

Preheat the oven to *200°C/180°C fan/gas mark 6*.

Heat the olive oil in a medium frying pan. Add the onion, rosemary, balsamic vinegar, Worcestershire sauce and date paste with a pinch of salt, and cook over a low-medium heat for a few minutes until the onions soften and start to brown.

Add the tomatoes, mustard, paprika and butter beans, and bring to a gentle boil for 15 minutes with the lid on, until the tomatoes have broken down. Add up to 100ml of water to thin the mixture if needed. If you are using Parmesan, stir through in the final minute of cooking.

Meanwhile, cut the top off the cob loaf and pull out the insides. Break the top and insides of the loaf into bite-sized pieces (these will be used to scoop into the bean mix). Drizzle the pieces with olive oil and seasoning before spreading out on a baking tray. Brush the outside of the cob loaf with some more olive oil and place it on a second baking tray. Place both trays in the oven for 10 minutes or until golden brown.

To serve, spoon the bean mixture into the hollowed-out cob loaf, and serve with the crunchy bread pieces and extra Parmesan (if using).

Storage   The beans will keep in the fridge for up to 3 days and up to 1 month in the freezer.

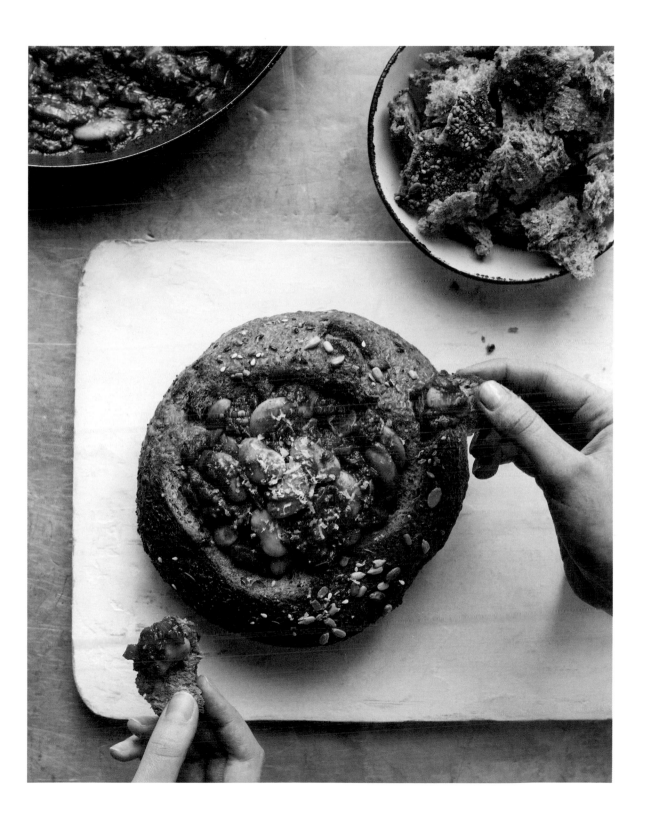

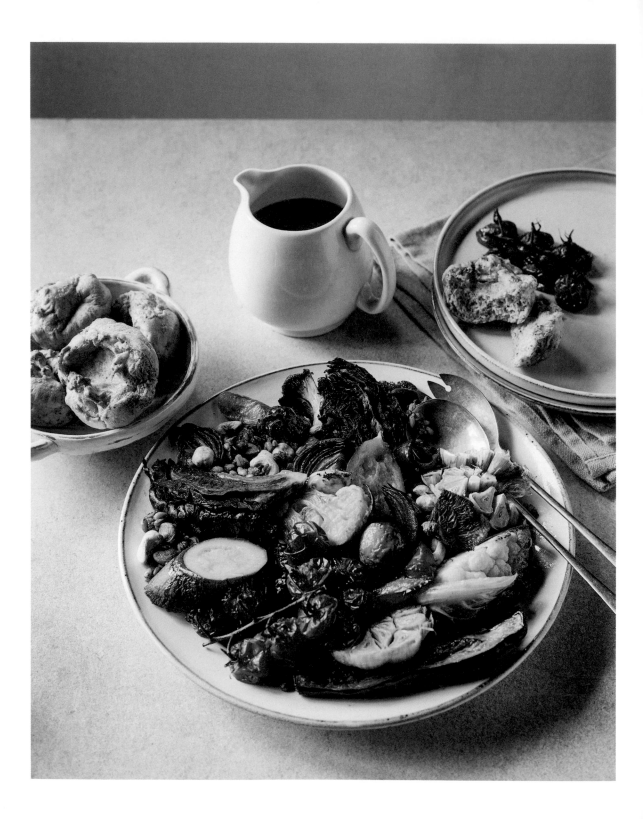

Rainbow roast with green Yorkshire puds

Plant Points
21.5

Serves **4 (with leftover veg to make the Moroccan couscous)**   Prep **20 mins**   Cook **55 mins**

 Fridge raid   **Freezer**

Sunday roasts never looked so colourful! Complete with Yorkshire pudding and gravy, this dish is not only gut-warming but also gives you a head start with your weekly plant points. I make a double batch most Sundays so that a supply of roast veg is ready for the week ahead.

Roast veg:
1 red onion, quartered
1 aubergine, quartered
½ cauliflower, quartered
1 large courgette, quartered
200g Brussels sprouts
1 pepper, quartered
2 carrots, halved
200g tomatoes, ideally on
    the vine
½ small cabbage, quartered
4 oyster mushrooms, or
    mushrooms of choice
1 whole unpeeled garlic, halved
    widthways
2 tbsp extra virgin olive oil

Toppers (optional):
250g precooked mixed
    wholegrains
80g mixed nuts, or nut of choice
2 tbsp mixed seeds

**Green Yorkshire puds
(makes 4–6):**
6 tsp sunflower oil (1 tsp per
    Yorkshire)
75g plain flour
2 large eggs
125ml soy milk, or milk of choice
15g baby spinach leaves
1 tbsp poppy seeds

To serve:
250ml wild mushroom gravy
    (page 270), or gravy of choice

Preheat the oven to *200°C/180°C/gas mark 6*. Get whichever veg you're using (you can use whatever you have in the fridge, I've just listed my favourites). Spread them across two large baking trays lined with non-stick baking paper. Drizzle with the olive oil, and place in the bottom two levels of the oven for around 50 minutes (turning the veg after 20 minutes).

Meanwhile, pour the sunflower oil for the Yorkshire puds into 4 muffin holes. When you turn the roast veg, place the muffin tray in the oven to heat up for 10 minutes. You want this to be really hot before you put in the batter.

While the oil is heating, place all the ingredients for the Yorkshires in a food processor (except for the poppy seeds) and blitz until the veg is well blended (approx. 1 minute). Then stir in the poppy seeds. Carefully remove the muffin tin from the oven and pour in the batter. Place the tin straight back in the oven and bake for 20–25 minutes. Although tempting, don't open the oven door during this time, as it will prevent them from rising.

Remove the Yorkshires from the oven. If the veg isn't quite done, add the mixed wholegrains, nuts and seeds and cook for 5 minutes. If the veg is ready, transfer to a plate and cover with foil. Spread the mixed wholegrains, nuts and seeds on the heated tray, and cook for 5 minutes or until lightly toasted.

Plate the roast veg and toppers, along with the Yorkshire puds. Pour on the wild mushroom gravy, or gravy of choice.

Tip Prefer a 'naked', aka gravy-free, roast? Cover your veg in one of these flavour options before roasting: 1–2 tsp za'atar, 1 tbsp rosemary and 1 tbsp thyme, or 1 tsp smoked paprika, along with a big pinch of rock salt and ground pepper.

Storage The leftover roast veg will keep in the fridge for 3 days, but I suggest using it up in my Moroccan couscous salad recipe (page 208). Cooked Yorkshires can be frozen for up to 1 month in an airtight container or a freezer bag. The gravy will keep in the fridge for 3 days or can be frozen for up to 1 month.

Barley butternut risotto

Serves **4** Prep **10 mins** Cook **40 mins**

 Fridge raid ✳ **Freezer**

There are few things more comforting than a bowl of creamy risotto. Switching up the wholegrain from rice to barley gives it a deliciously nutty taste (not to mention the added fibre, boasting 13g per portion) – and you can mix up the other plants to suit what's in season or what you have in the fridge.

2 tbsp extra virgin olive oil
1 leek, sliced (approx. 150g)
3 celery sticks, sliced (approx. 130g)
½ butternut squash or sweet potato,
    diced (approx. 400g)
3 garlic cloves, grated or crushed
    (approx. 12g)
8 sage leaves or ½ tsp dried sage
240g pearl barley
900ml vegetable stock
30g Parmesan, grated
150g spring greens or spinach, chopped

To serve (optional):
extra virgin olive oil, for frying
4 sage leaves
2 tbsp pumpkin seeds
20g Parmesan, shaved
lemon zest, to taste

Add the olive oil to a large cast-iron casserole pot or saucepan and place over a medium heat. Add the leek, celery and butternut squash and cook for 10 minutes, stirring occasionally until starting to soften.

Then stir in the garlic and sage, and cook for 1 minute before adding the pearl barley and vegetable stock. Bring up to a gentle boil and cook for 30 minutes with the lid off or until the pearl barley is al dente.

Stir the pot every 10 minutes or so in between your de-stressing exercise (see page 116) to make sure nothing catches. Add a splash of water if it gets too dry.

Stir in the grated Parmesan, followed by the spring greens. Cook until the greens are just wilted (approx. 3–4 minutes). Season to taste.

If you want to really impress and add an extra plant point, serve with some crispy sage leaves and pumpkin seeds. To achieve this, heat a splash of olive oil in a frying pan and, when hot, drop in the sage leaves and pumpkin seeds and fry for a minute until crisp.

You can also serve the barley risotto with Parmesan shavings and lemon zest.

Storage This can be kept in the fridge for 3 days, or frozen (minus the greens) for up to 1 month.

Switch To make this 100 per cent plant-based, simply switch Parmesan out for 2 tbsp nutritional yeast or more to taste.

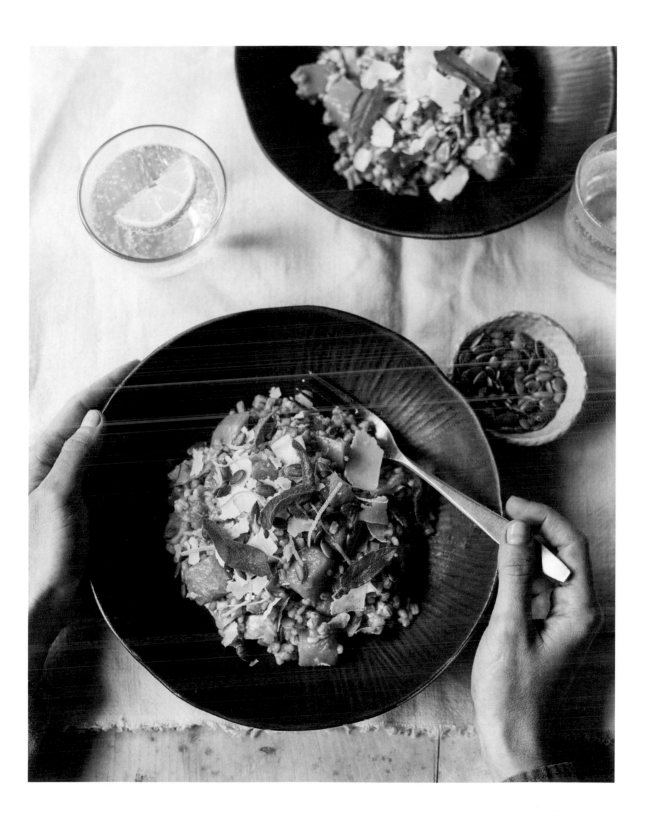

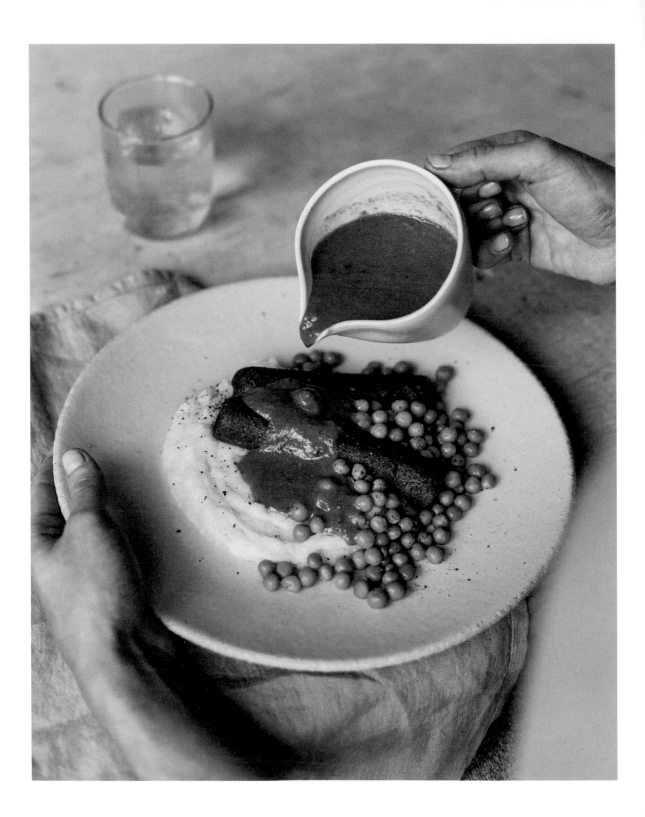

Bangers and mash revamped

Serves **4**   Prep **15 mins, plus chilling**   Cook **20 mins**

 Freezer

A plant twist on a classic. Creamy prebiotic mash topped with meaty plant-sausages and a pop of freshness from the peas, drizzled with mouth-watering gravy – this one will be a family favourite.

2–3 slices seeded bread (approx. 100g)

2 tbsp ground flaxseed (approx. 10g)

1 large aubergine, roughly chopped (approx. 400g)

120g white mushrooms or mushrooms of choice, roughly chopped

1 apple (approx. 120g), roughly chopped

3 tbsp extra virgin olive oil

1 tbsp dried oregano

2 tbsp Worcestershire sauce

15g parsley, finely chopped

1 x 200g tin of green lentils, drained and rinsed

To serve:

320g peas, fresh or frozen

creamy mash and wild mushroom gravy (see page 270 for recipe)

To make the sausages, blitz the bread and flaxseed together in a food processor until they form a course flour (approx. 30–45 seconds), then tip into a bowl. Add the aubergine, mushrooms and apple to the food processor and pulse until roughly chopped.

Heat 1 tbsp of olive oil in a frying pan on a medium-high heat, and add the aubergine mix from the food processor, along with the oregano and Worcestershire sauce. Fry until the liquid from the veg has reduced and the mix has softened (it should take approx. 10 minutes). Season to taste, then tip back into the food processor with the parsley, lentils and bread mix, and roughly blitz for 30 seconds.

Chill the mix in the fridge for at least 10 minutes to firm up while you prep the mash and gravy.

Divide the sausage mix into 10. Roll each portion into a sausage shape. Heat 2 tbsp of olive oil in the frying pan. Add the sausages and cook for 10 minutes over a low heat, turning gently until golden all over and hot through.

Cook the peas following pack instructions, and serve with the sausages, mash and gravy.

Storage The uncooked sausage mix will keep in the fridge for up to 2 days and can be frozen for up to 2 months.

Tip The sausage mix is also delicious when made into falafel-like patties and served in a pitta with pickles and yoghurt.

Chicken 'n' veg meaty balls

Plant Points 4.75

Serves **4 (28 meatballs, plus leftover to make the *reinvented* chicken burgers)**

Prep **15 mins**   Cook **20 mins**

 FODMAP Lite   **Freezer**

All of the succulent chicken flavour with just half the meat, and a great way to introduce more veg to a meat-loving palate. Versatility is the name of these juicy meatballs' game – you could bake them and enjoy with a salad, add to a stir fry or your favourite soup, but my favourite is to drizzle them with hoisin sauce and serve on a bed of quinoa rice (page 271). Plus, the leftover mixture can be turned into a burger recipe (page 205).

4–5 slices seeded bread, or bread of choice (approx. 160g)
500g boneless chicken thighs
15g ginger, peeled and sliced
1 tsp sea salt
1 green pepper, roughly chopped (approx. 165g prepped)
1 carrot, roughly chopped (approx. 85g prepped)
30g fresh coriander, roughly chopped
6 spring onions, roughly chopped (approx. 50g prepped)
1 large egg, beaten
extra virgin olive oil, for drizzling and frying

Preheat the oven to *190°C/170°C fan/gas mark 5*.

Blitz the bread to crumbs in a food processor for around 15 seconds, then place in a bowl to one side.

Place the chicken, ginger and salt in the food processor and whizz until smooth, for approx. 1 minute. Add the pepper and carrot, and pulse about 5 times until the veg is all finely chopped but still visible. You may need to scrape the sides down. Next, add the coriander and spring onions, and pulse a couple of times until chopped.

Add in the egg and breadcrumbs, and pulse until just mixed. Set aside 230g for the burger recipe (if making) and divide the rest into 28 meatballs (approx. 25g each).

Spread out on a baking tray lined with non-stick baking paper, drizzle with olive oil and bake for 15 minutes. To make golden brown, finish in a frying pan over medium heat with olive oil for 5 minutes.

Plate with the quinoa rice from page 271 or your favourite sides.

Storage The uncooked balls/burgers can be made 24 hours in advance and stored in the fridge ready to cook, or frozen for up to 3 months in an airtight container. Defrost overnight and cook following the recipe instructions.

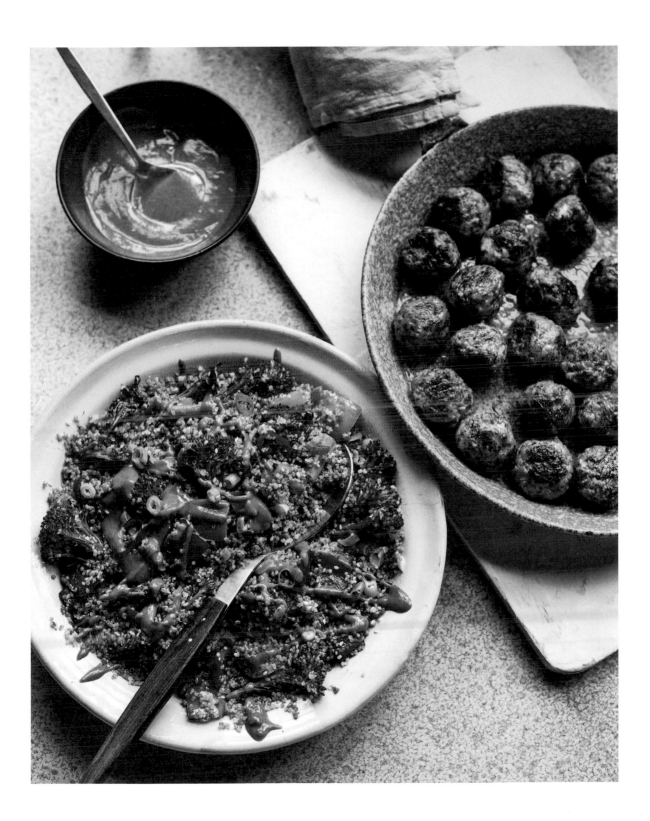

Sides

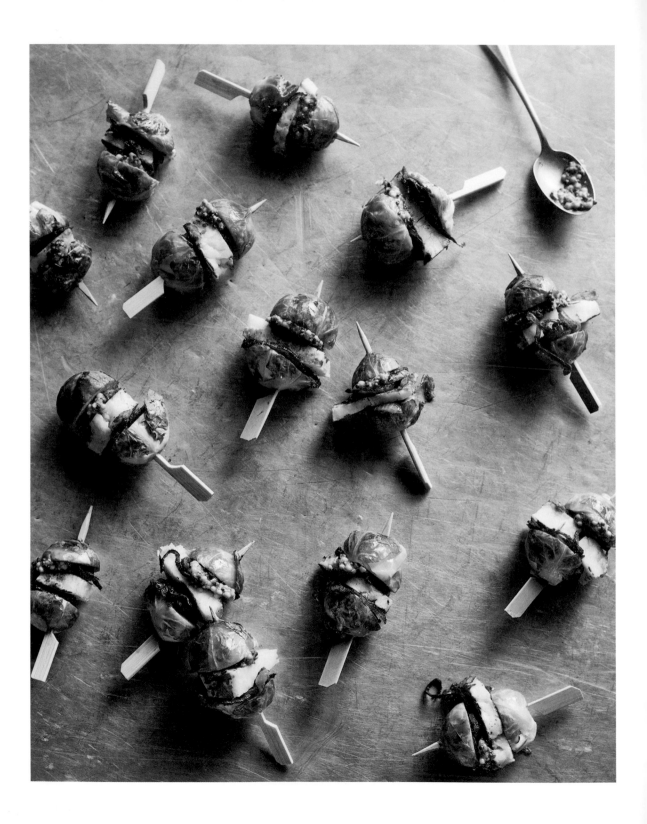

Halloumi sprout bites

Makes **15 bites**   Prep **20 mins**   Cook **20 mins**

If you're not big on Brussels sprouts, let me change your mind! Delicious roasted, the sweet-and-sour sticky onions and salty halloumi take them to the next level. Oh, and did you know sprouts and onions are both good sources of prebiotics too?

15 large Brussels sprouts (approx. 380g)
½ tbsp extra virgin olive oil
80g halloumi, cut into 5 slices
1 tbsp wholegrain mustard

Caramelized onions:
1 tbsp extra virgin olive oil
1 red onion, thinly sliced (approx. 150g)
1 tbsp balsamic vinegar
1 Medjool date, made into a paste (see page 134), or 1 tbsp sweetener

cocktail sticks

Preheat the oven to *200°C/180°C fan/gas mark 6.*

Line a baking tray with non-stick baking paper. Toss the sprouts in olive oil and a pinch of seasoning, spread out on the tray and bake for 12–15 minutes until just cooked and starting to take on a little colour.

Meanwhile, in a medium frying pan, heat 1 tbsp of olive oil over a medium heat before adding the caramelized onion ingredients (onion, balsamic vinegar and date paste). Cook for 15 minutes (or longer if you have time), stirring frequently until sticky and caramelized.

In a small frying pan over a medium heat, fry the halloumi for 1–2 minutes on each side until golden. Remove from the pan and put to one side.

To assemble, cut each slice of halloumi into 3 pieces. Cut each sprout in half. Place each half on a cocktail stick, add some onion, and hold in place with a piece of halloumi. Add a little more onion, a little drop of the mustard, and top with the other half of the sprout. Repeat until all are assembled, and enjoy!

Storage Will keep for 3 days in the fridge.

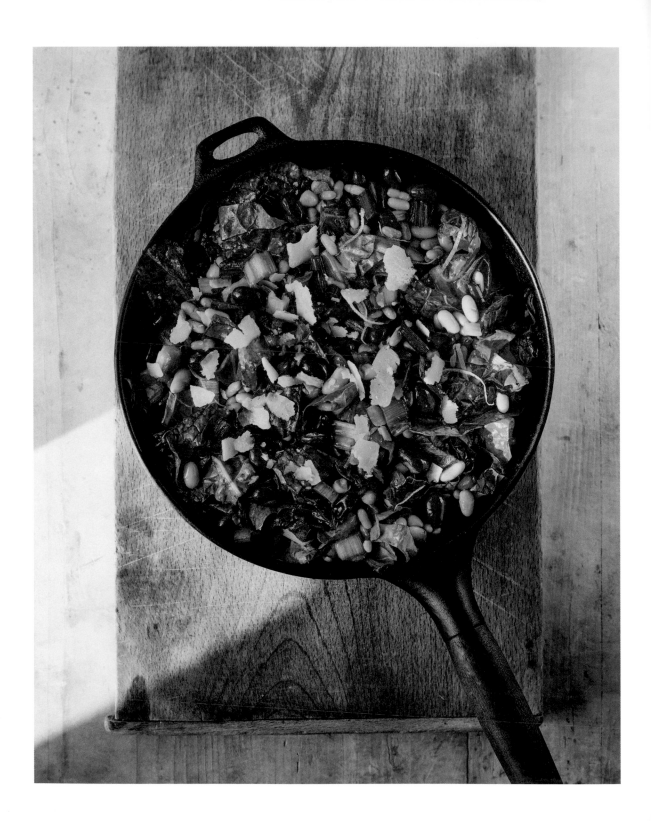

Greens and beans

Plant Points
3.5

Serves **6**   Prep **5 mins**   Cook **5 mins**

 FODMAP Lite   **Fridge raid**   **Zero waste**

My top fibre and diversity tip: add a side of veg or beans to whatever you're having (including your Saturday night take-out!). This quick and easy dish is the ideal way to do just that, packing in 10g of fibre per portion. It's the perfect example of how a little seasoning and light cooking can transform a humble tin of beans and greens into a stunningly simple but tasty side in 10 minutes flat.

2 tbsp extra virgin olive oil

2 garlic cloves, grated (approx. 8g)

300g Swiss chard, stalks finely chopped and leaves roughly chopped, or greens of choice (e.g pak choi, spinach, collard greens)

1 x 400g tin of cannellini beans, drained and rinsed

1 x 400g tin of red kidney beans, drained and rinsed

zest of 1 lemon (approx. 5g), to taste

½ tbsp soy sauce

40g Parmesan, grated

In a frying pan, heat the olive oil and garlic for a minute, before sautéing the trimmed greens. After a few minutes add the tinned beans, lemon zest and soy sauce. Serve straight out of the pan with some grated Parmesan.

Switch Up for the diversity challenge? Swap the greens for a packet of stir-fry mixed veg.

Sticky parsnips

Plant Points
5.5

Serves **4**   Prep **5 mins**   Cook **15 mins**

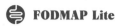 **FODMAP Lite**

Not a fan of parsnips? Neither was I, until I discovered I just wasn't dressing them right. The sticky marinade really elevates the humble parsnip to something centre-stage (pictured on page 227). And it gets even better for busy people as the marinade has a dual role, coating the parsnips and marinating the orange-glazed roasted salmon on page 226.

750g parsnips, washed
sesame oil, for frying

Marinade:
juice of 1 orange (approx. 80ml)
2 garlic cloves, grated or minced
20g ginger, grated
3 tbsp soy sauce
3 tbsp mirin
1 tbsp sesame oil
2 Medjool dates, made into a paste (see
    page 134), or 2 tbsp sweetener
1 tbsp wholemeal flour, and additional
    for coating

Toppers (optional):
1 tbsp sesame seeds
1 spring onion, finely chopped

Top and tail the parsnips and cut into bite-size cubes. Steam on the hob for 10 minutes or microwave for 7 minutes with a splash of water.

Meanwhile, place all the ingredients for the marinade (except for the flour) in a small saucepan, bring to the boil and then simmer for 5–10 minutes until reduced and syrupy. Remove from the heat and slowly sprinkle in the flour as you stir rapidly – this will prevent clumps from forming. Roll the parsnips in flour before coating with the thickened marinade.

Add a layer of sesame oil to a frying pan on a medium-high heat, then add the coated parsnips. Fry for 1–2 minutes on each side or until golden brown. Keep your eye on them while they are frying, as the parsnips can burn easily.

Once ready to serve, sprinkle with the sesame seeds and spring onion. Best enjoyed hot from the pan.

Storage   Keeps in the fridge for up to 3 days.

Veg all-dressed-up

Plant Points
6.75

Serves **4 as a side, or 2 for a light meal**   Prep **10 mins**   Cook **5 mins**

 FODMAP Lite   **Fridge raid**

Gone are the days of forcing down boring veg. This recipe shows how, with just a simple dressing, plain steamed veg can be transformed into a side you actually crave. Served in a fun edible bowl that not just kids will love.

400g bag of prepared mixed veg
4 small wholemeal wraps, or wraps
 of choice

Avocado pesto:
½ ripe avocado (approx. 60g flesh)
5g fresh basil
40ml extra virgin olive oil
½ garlic clove (approx. 2–3g)
25g pine nuts
2 tbsp grated Parmesan or
 nutritional yeast

Creamy cashew:
50ml live thick yoghurt
1 tsp Dijon mustard
juice of ½ small lemon (approx. 15ml)
50g natural cashews
2 tbsp extra virgin olive oil

Preheat the oven to *200°C/180°C fan/gas mark 6*. Turn a muffin tin over and tuck the wraps into the gaps to make diamond-shaped edible bowls. Bake in the oven for 5 minutes, then set aside to cool.

Meanwhile, cook the mixed veg in the microwave according to packet instructions (usually by piercing the bag and cooking for approx. 3–4 minutes). Alternatively, open the packet and steam the veg over a saucepan of simmering water for 3–4 minutes.

For the avocado pesto option, use a hand blender to blitz the ingredients together until you have a thick pesto. This should take approx. 2 minutes. Season with sea salt and black pepper to taste.

For the creamy cashew option, use a small food processor to blitz the ingredients together until you have a thick sauce. This should take approx. 2 minutes. If it's too thick to pour, add a splash of hot water to thin. Season with sea salt and black pepper to taste.

Assemble the veg in the edible bowl, and dollop on the avocado pesto or creamy cashew sauce.

Storage   Both dressings keep in the fridge for up to 3 days. I use the leftovers as dips, spreads and even pasta sauce – they're so versatile!

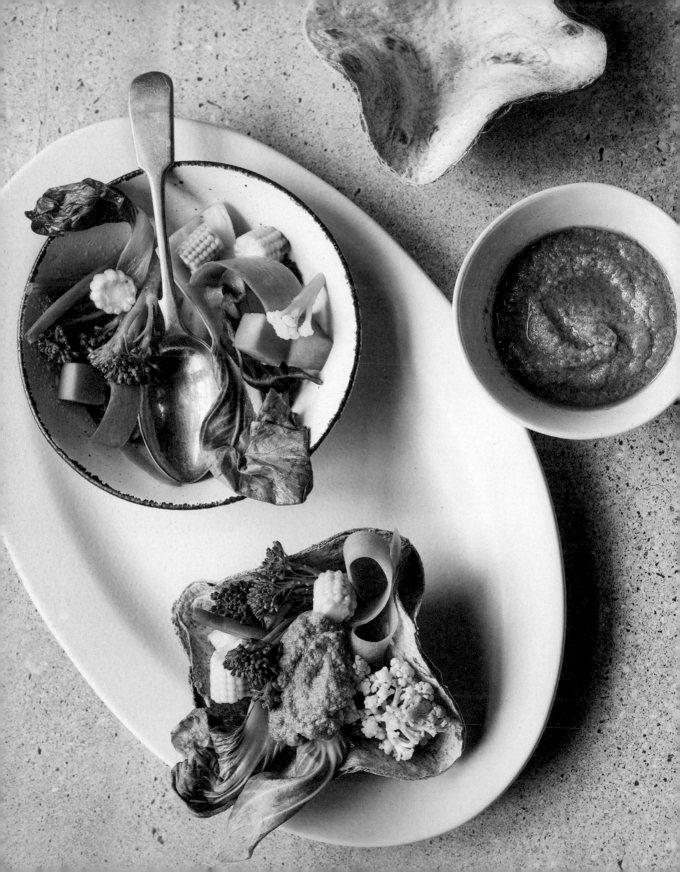

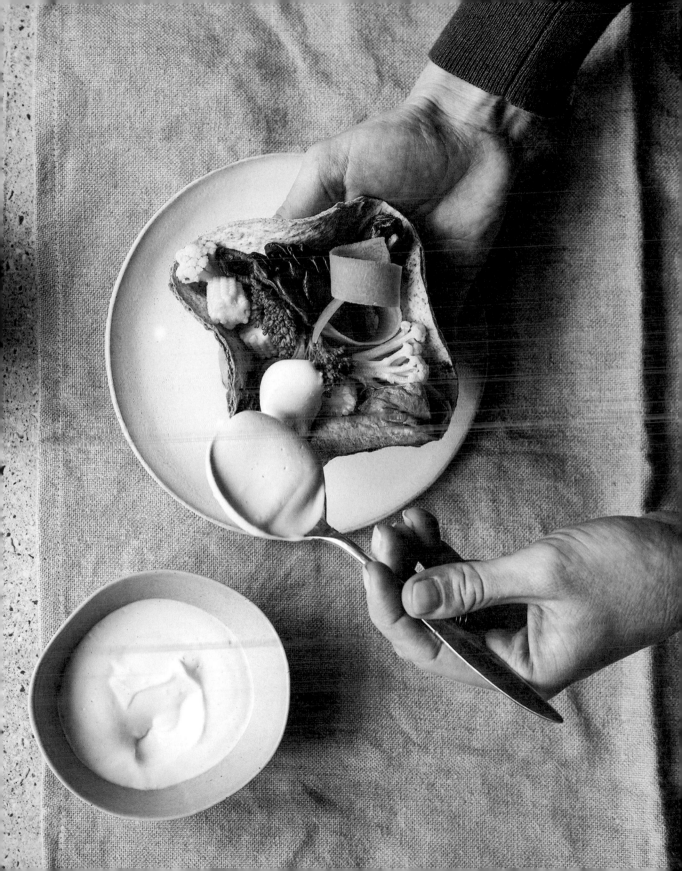

Spinach balls with tahini sauce

Makes **20 bites**   Prep **15 mins**   Cook **5 mins**

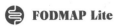 **FODMAP Lite**

Inspired by the Japanese dish spinach gomae, this is a tasty way to get in your greens. Despite being packed full of phytochemicals and fibre, the tahini dipping sauce will ensure those who aren't yet great with greens won't suspect a thing.

400g baby spinach leaves, washed
1 tsp sesame oil

Tahini dipping sauce:
1 tsp soy sauce or more to taste
2 Medjool dates, made into a paste (see page 134), or 2 tbsp sweetener
juice of 1 lemon (approx. 50ml), to taste
¼ cup tahini
1 tsp sesame oil

Topper:
½ tbsp sesame seeds, toasted
tooth picks (optional)

Place the spinach in a large saucepan over a medium heat with the lid on. Allow to steam and wilt for 3–4 minutes. Rinse immediately under cold water and squeeze out any excess water, first with your hands and then in a clean cloth for the final squeeze. Place in a bowl and toss the sesame oil through.

To make the spinach balls, divide the spinach into 20 portions and shape into balls. Try to keep some of the leaves whole to wrap around each ball to hold it together. Keep to one side on a piece of kitchen towel, to help absorb any excess liquid.

Place the ingredients for the dipping sauce in a jug and blitz with a hand blender until smooth. Taste to check the balance of sweet, salty and sour, adding a little more lemon juice or soy sauce as needed. If the dip is a little thick, add a dash of water until it reaches your preferred consistency.

Transfer the spinach balls to a plate and scatter the sesame seeds on top. Serve with the dipping sauce and optional tooth picks.

Storage   Dipping sauces keep for up to 1 week in the fridge.

Tip   If you can't find toasted sesame seeds, make your own. Heat a small non-stick frying pan over a low heat. Add the sesame seeds and fry for 1–2 minutes, stirring constantly until lightly golden, then tip on to a plate.

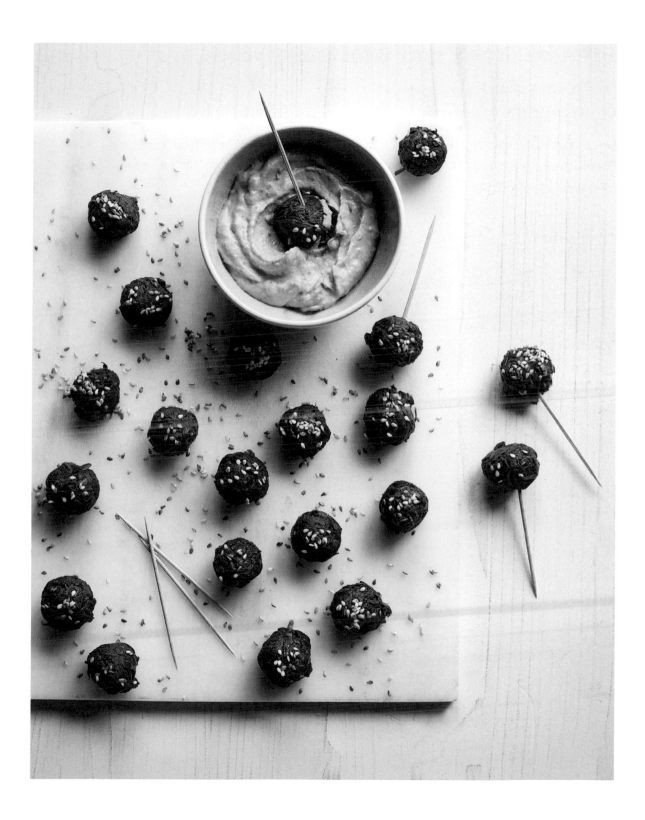

Creamy mash and wild mushroom gravy

Plant Points 7.5

Serves **4**   Prep **15 mins**   Cook **25 mins**

 Freezer   **Zero waste**

Gone are the days of single-plant-point mash. This smooth and fluffy celeriac and cauliflower mash, giving you triple plant points, is really brought to life with the wild mushroom gravy (pictured on page 254). A match made in mash heaven.

Creamy mash:
450g floury potato (such as Maris Piper), peeled and cut into 4cm chunks
250g celeriac, peeled and cut into 3cm chunks
250g cauliflower florets
2 tsp extra virgin olive oil
25g finely grated Parmesan, or more to taste
1 tsp Dijon mustard

Wild mushroom gravy (makes 250ml):
600ml vegetable stock
15g dried porcini mushrooms
1 tbsp olive oil
100g frozen sofrito vegetable mix (or 35g each of carrot, onions and celery, chopped)
1 tbsp red miso paste, or white miso
2 tbsp wholemeal flour, or flour of choice

Add the potato and celeriac to a saucepan of boiling water and cook for 10 minutes. Add the cauliflower and cook for a further 5–10 minutes, or until soft. Drain and leave to dry for a few minutes, while you make the gravy.

For the gravy, add the boiling water to the vegetable stock, along with the dried mushrooms. Allow to soak for 15 minutes.

Once the veg has cooled, blitz together with a hand blender until smooth (approx. 1 minute). Return the saucepan to a low heat and cook for 5 minutes, stirring frequently to simmer off any liquid from the veg. Take off the heat before stirring in the olive oil, Parmesan and the Dijon mustard. Season to taste, and cover to keep warm.

Meanwhile, heat the olive oil for the gravy in a frying pan. Add the sofrito mix and cook for 5 minutes over a medium heat, until softened and starting to take on some colour.

Strain the stock, before adding it to a blender, along with the vegetable mix, miso paste and flour. Blend until smooth (approx. 1 minute).

Finally return the gravy to the saucepan and simmer for 10 minutes until thickened, stirring regularly.

Serve with bangers (for recipe see page 255) or other protein of choice.

Storage   The gravy freezes well for up to 3 months, so you could double the quantity and freeze half. Keeps in the fridge for up to 3 days.

Tip   Love a chunky gravy? Keep in half the porcini mushrooms and blend. Add any leftover mushrooms to your next stir fry. Don't throw them out!

Quinoa rice with hoisin drizzle

Plant Points
7.75

Serves **4**   Prep **10 mins**   Cook **7 mins**

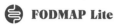 FODMAP Lite

When you taste this flavourful and fibre-filled rice alternative, you'll wonder why you hadn't swapped out the bland white stuff sooner. Not only does it add more texture, but it soaks up the sweet and salty hoisin drizzle perfectly (pictured on page 257). Enjoy it with the chicken 'n' veg meaty balls from page 256.

½ tbsp extra virgin olive oil
2 peppers (approx. 190 g), diced
1 large red chilli (approx. 14g), sliced
100g Tenderstem broccoli, chopped
400g precooked quinoa (or 150g uncooked, cooked to packet instructions)
2 spring onions, sliced (approx. 20g)
2 tsp sesame seeds (optional)

Hoisin drizzle:
¼ cup soy sauce
2 tbsp peanut butter
1 Medjool date, made into a paste (see page 134), or 1 tbsp sweetener
1 tsp balsamic vinegar
2 tsp sesame oil
1 small clove garlic, grated or minced (approx. 2g)
½ teaspoon red miso paste

Blitz all the ingredients for the hoisin drizzle together in a high-speed blender.

Heat the olive oil in a large frying pan or wok. Add the peppers, chilli and broccoli, and cook for 3–4 minutes until just starting to take on some colour.

Add the quinoa and season to taste. Cook for another 2–3 minutes until the quinoa is hot through, then stir in the spring onions and sesame seeds (if using).

Drizzle the sauce over the quinoa rice and serve alongside the chicken balls or protein of choice.

Tip For added diversity, choose a multicoloured pack of peppers. This dish also works well with red rice.

Storage Leftover hoisin drizzle will keep in a jar for up to 2 weeks in the fridge.

Desserts

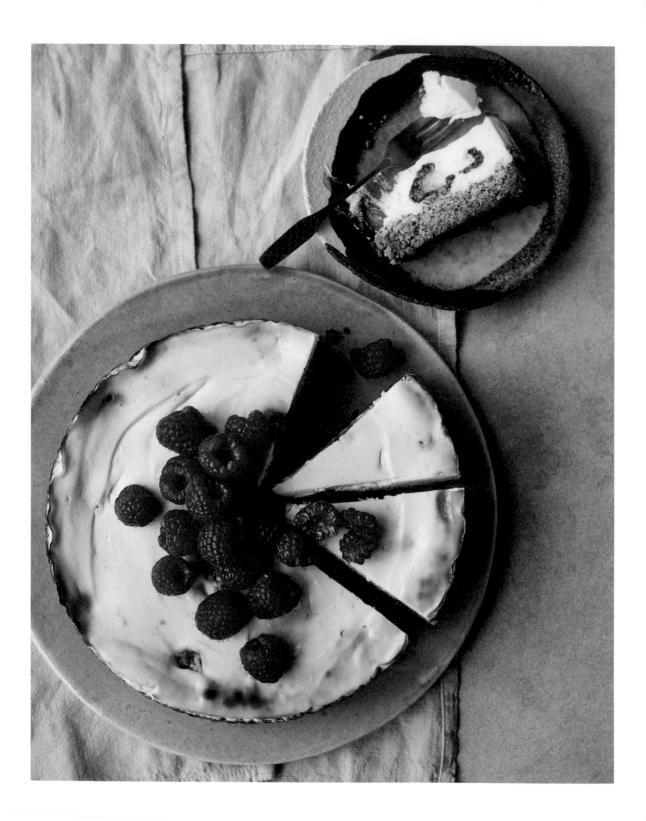

Raspberry and lemon ricotta baked cheesecake

Makes **12 slices**   Prep **15 mins**   Cook **1 hour, plus chilling**

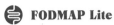 **FODMAP Lite**

I love cheesecake, but shop-bought versions can be notoriously high in saturated fat. This creamy cheesecake is a gut-loving treat, with fermented dairy, bursts of colour from the juicy berries, and a deliciously nutty base that's just sweet enough.

Base:
100g cooked quinoa
200g walnuts
6 Medjool dates, pitted (approx. 100g)
1 tbsp ground ginger (optional)
1 large egg, lightly beaten

Cheesecake:
500g ricotta
200g live thick yoghurt
2 large eggs, plus 1 egg yolk (use the
    leftover white in tomorrow's omelette
    bowl, see page 139)
3 tbsp honey, or sweetener of choice
3 tbsp plain flour
juice of 1 lemon (approx. 45ml), plus zest
150g frozen raspberries

Topper (optional):
100g fresh raspberries

Preheat the oven to *190°C/170°C fan/gas mark 5*, and line the base and sides of a 20cm high-sided spring-form cake tin with non-stick baking paper.

Place the quinoa, walnuts, dates and ground ginger in a food processor and blitz until combined (approx. 30–60 seconds), leaving some texture in the crumb. Stir in the egg.

Tip into the lined cake tin and press down in an even layer. Place in the preheated oven and bake for 20 minutes.

Meanwhile, place all the cheesecake ingredients, except the frozen berries, in a food processor and blitz to combine for approx. 1 minute. Scrape the sides and blitz again for another minute.

When the base has been in the oven for 20 minutes, take it out and pour the cheesecake mix on top, and dot in the frozen berries as you go.

Turn the oven down to *180°C/160°C/gas mark 4*, and return the cake tin to the oven. Bake for 40 minutes until the middle has just set. If there is still any wobble, give it another 5–10 minutes.

Turn the oven off, crack the door open and allow the cake to cool in the oven. Then remove and chill in the fridge overnight before serving with fresh berries.

Storage Best eaten soon after it's chilled, but keeps up to 5 days in an airtight container in the fridge.

Switch Already had raspberries this week? Swap for blueberries.

Trail mix loaf cake with yoghurt and white chocolate glaze

Makes **12 slices**   Prep **15 mins**   Cook **40 mins**

 FODMAP Lite   **Freezer**

My gut-loving take on a traditional fruit cake. Not only is it quick and easy to make for those on a tight schedule, unlike boring fruit cakes, the diverse mix of textures and flavours will have you going back for seconds. Ideal as an afternoon treat to share with friends and family, or drop the glaze and have it as a snack-on-the-go to fuel those busy days.

3 large eggs
1 tsp vanilla extract
4 very ripe bananas (approx. 400g)
200g wholemeal flour
2 tsp baking powder
100g walnuts, roughly chopped
70g dried figs, roughly chopped
50g dried mango, chopped
1 tbsp mixed seeds
50g almonds, chopped
1 raw beetroot, coarsely grated
   (approx. 100g)

Glaze:
100g white chocolate
50g live thick yoghurt

Preheat the oven to *190°C/170°C fan/gas mark 5* and line a 900g (2lb) loaf tin with non-stick baking paper.

In a food processor blend together the eggs, vanilla extract and bananas until combined (approx. 1 minute).

In a large bowl, mix the flour and baking powder, followed by the walnuts, figs, mango, seeds, almonds and beetroot. Pour in the wet ingredients, and fold in.

Pour the mixture into the prepared tin and bake for 40 minutes, or until a skewer comes out clean. Allow the cake to cool in the tin on a wire rack before removing.

To make the glaze, first melt the chocolate. Add the chocolate to a heatproof mixing bowl and either place over a pan of simmering water to melt, or heat in the microwave in 30-second bursts, stirring in between.

Mix the yoghurt into the melted chocolate and spread over the cake.

Storage   The cake (without the glaze) can be kept in an airtight container in the fridge for 5 days. It can also be frozen, wrapped in cling film, for up to 1 month.

Cream-less ice cream – two ways

 FODMAP Lite   **Freezer**

Whose freezer wouldn't benefit from a tub of gut-loving ice cream? You certainly don't need a special ice-cream machine – or even cream or added sugar – to make an indulgent and smooth dessert. For those of you who love experimenting (or encouraging the kids to eat their greens!), the hidden-veg version is for you; and for those short on time, jump straight to the no-freeze option.

Plant Points
9.5

Hidden-veg option

Serves **4**   Prep **15 mins, plus freezing time**   Cook **2 mins (if using cabbage)**

80g sweetheart cabbage, shredded, steamed and cooled (optional)

2 large very ripe bananas, roughly chopped and frozen (approx. 240g weight)

200g tinned full-fat coconut milk, frozen

½ avocado (approx. 80g flesh)

3 Medjool dates, pitted and roughly chopped (approx. 50g)

10g baby spinach leaves

Optional fillings (choose one):

100g chickpea cookie dough (see page 163 for recipe)

2g mint leaves and 50g dark chocolate chips, roughly chopped

To steam the cabbage, fill a steamer with 2cm of water and bring to the boil. Place the shredded cabbage in the basket, put the lid on and steam for 5 minutes until soft. Alternatively, add a little water to a microwave-safe dish and microwave for 2 minutes on high, or until the cabbage has softened. Place in the freezer for a few minutes to chill completely.

Take the frozen banana and coconut milk out of the freezer 5 minutes before you want to make the ice cream: this will make it easier to blend. Cut the frozen coconut milk into small chunks and pop into a high-powered blender along with the banana. Blitz for 5 minutes until the ice crystals have broken down – it will look like slushy snow

Add the avocado, dates, steamed cabbage and spinach. Blitz for another 4–5 minutes until smooth – you may need to stop and scrape down the sides occasionally.

If using fillings, blitz the mint through the ice cream for a few seconds and stir through the choc chips, or alternatively stir in chunks of the chickpea cookie dough.

Decant the ice cream into a 1-litre airtight tub as quickly as you can to limit the melting, and place it in the freezer for at least 4 hours to firm up.

No-freeze option

Serves **4**   Prep **5 mins (plus freezing time)**

400g frozen blueberries, or
   berry of choice
400g live thick yoghurt
2 very ripe bananas, frozen
   (approx. 200g)

Blitz together the berries, banana and yoghurt in a high-powered blender until smooth (approx. 1 minute) and you're done! Serve and enjoy.

Storage Can be frozen in an airtight container for up to 1 month.

Tip Chill the tub in the freezer while you're making the ice cream so it's cold when you pour the ice-cream mix in. This will help prevent the mix from melting, which will result in a creamier ice cream.

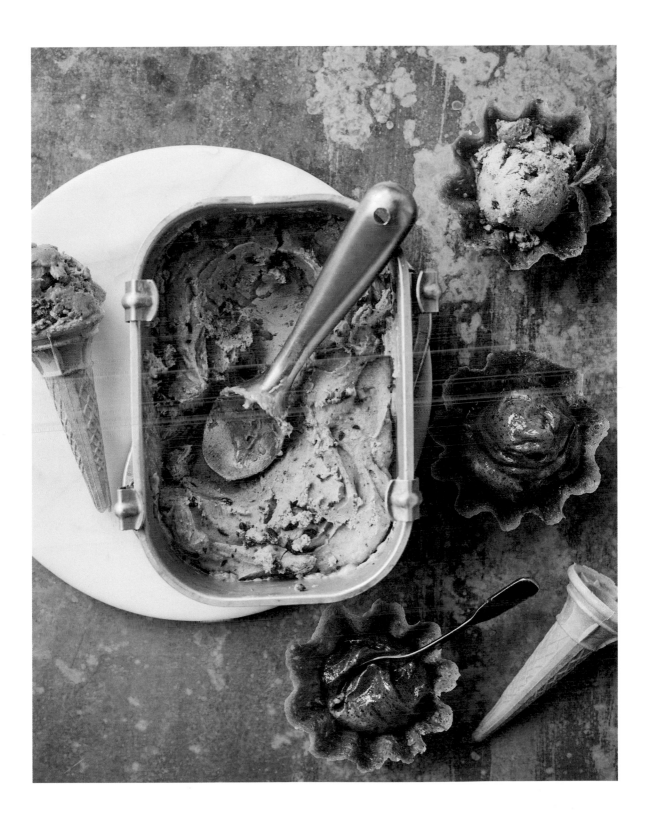

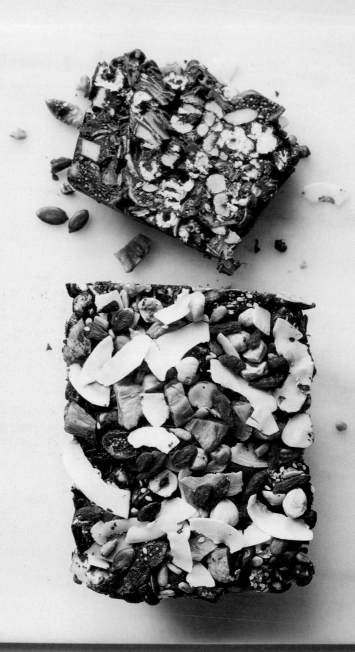

Prebiotic rocky road

Makes **15 slices**   Prep **15 mins, plus setting time**   Cook **5 mins**

 FODMAP Lite   **Zero waste**

With the combination of melt-in-your-mouth chocolate, crunchy nuts, chewy fruit and fluffy popcorn, this gut-loving treat trumps your standard rocky road on flavour. Your gut microbes will get quite the feast of phytochemicals, prebiotics and 5g of fibre per slice, using just store-cupboard ingredients. Plus, the cocoa flavanols in dark chocolate could even boost your brain power!

300g dark chocolate (min. 70%)
1 tbsp extra virgin olive oil, plus extra for popping corn

Toppers:
30g corn kernels, or natural popcorn
100g hazelnuts, chopped in half
50g brazil nuts, roughly chopped
2 tbsp mixed seeds
50g goji berries
30g coconut flakes
90g dried mango, chopped
90g dried figs, chopped

Toast the hazelnuts. Heat the oven to *200°C/180°C fan/gas mark 6* and place the nuts on a baking tray. Bake for 5 minutes, then remove and set aside to cool.

To pop the corn, heat a splash of olive oil in a saucepan over a medium heat. Add the corn kernels and shake gently to cover them in the oil. Put the lid on and the corn will start popping after a couple of minutes. Shake the saucepan occasionally to prevent burning. The corn should have finished popping after approx. 3–5 minutes.

Pour the popcorn into a large bowl and mix with all the ingredients apart from the chocolate, reserving a handful of the goji berries, mango, nuts and coconut flakes to decorate the top of the rocky road.

Break the chocolate into pieces and place in a heatproof mixing bowl. Either place over a saucepan of simmering water to melt or heat in the microwave in 30-second bursts, stirring in between. Stir in the 1 tbsp of olive oil, before pouring over the dry ingredients and mixing everything together well.

Line a 900g (2lb) loaf tin with non-stick baking paper, then pour the mixture into the tin. Scatter the reserved dry ingredients on top and press down. Place in the fridge to set (approx. 4 hours).

Once set, pull the rocky road out of the tin using the baking paper, and with a sharp knife cut into 15 slices and store in an airtight container in the fridge.

Storage Keeps for up to 2 weeks in the fridge in a sealed container.

Tip If you love ginger, add ¼–½ tsp of fresh grated ginger to the mix.

Switch Already had the listed dried fruits and nuts this week? Swap in any others you fancy.

Pistachio berry bursts

Makes **40 pieces**   Prep **25 mins, plus setting time**

 FODMAP Lite   **Freezer**

I must say, I'm quite proud of this one. It combines three of my favourite things: prebiotic pistachios, raspberries and white chocolate, all packed into little bursts of joy – and I'd argue even more aesthetically pleasing than your standard box of chocolates. Want to impress a friend (and their gut microbes)? Make these!

80g pistachios
1 tsp extra virgin olive oil
½ tsp vanilla extract
80g white chocolate
40 plump raspberries (approx. 180g)

Topper (optional):
80g dark chocolate

Blitz the pistachios, olive oil and vanilla in a small food processor for approx. 3 minutes, until a paste forms. You may need to scrape down the sides occasionally. Transfer into a mixing bowl.

Break the white chocolate into pieces and place in a heatproof mixing bowl. Either place over a saucepan of simmering water to melt or heat in the microwave in 30-second bursts, stirring in between. When melted, pour in with the pistachios and mix to form a dough.

Fill each raspberry with the mix, using clean fingers or a piping bag, so that the top of the raspberries are domed with the pistachio filling. Once filled, place in the fridge for a few minutes to set.

Meanwhile, break the dark chocolate into pieces (if using) and melt, using the same method as with the white chocolate.

Line a tray with non-stick baking paper, then carefully dip each filled raspberry in the melted chocolate using 2 teaspoons, or just your fingers. You can dip just the domed pistachio top, like an ice cream, or completely cover them – or do a mix of both.

Place on the tray in the fridge for 30 minutes to set before tucking in.

Storage The filled raspberries keep for 3 days in the fridge or up to 1 month in the freezer, although I doubt they'll last that long. The pistachio filling on its own keeps for a couple of weeks in a small sealed jar in the fridge, and is delicious spread on apple or pear slices. Such a treat!

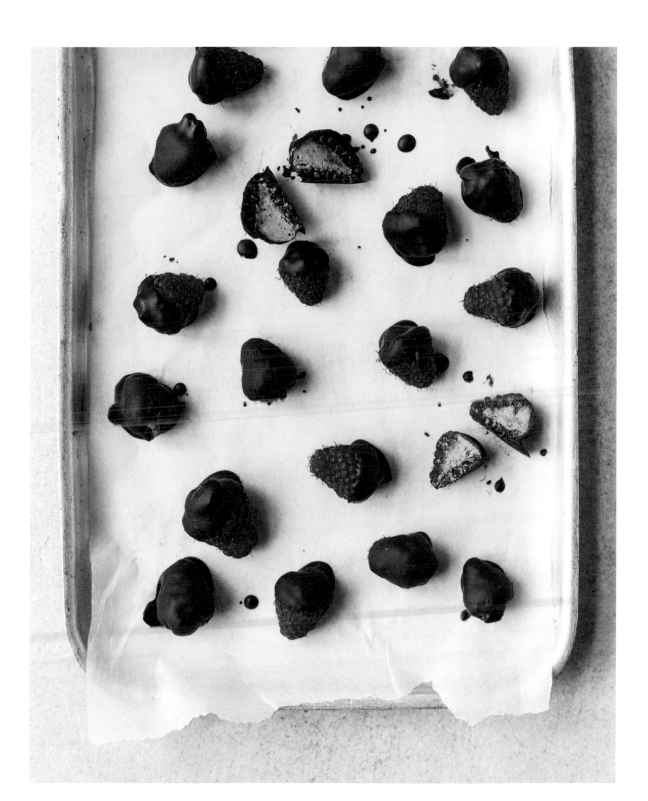

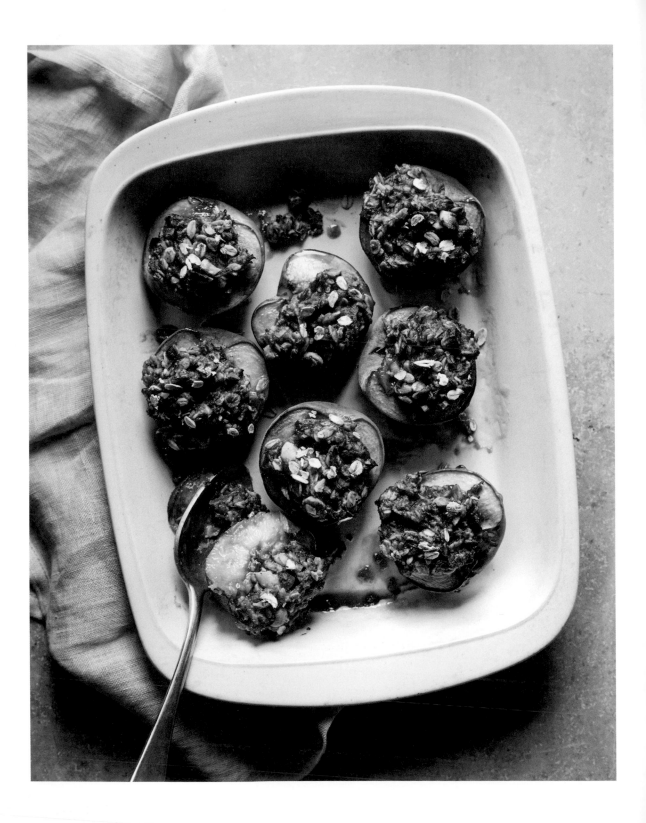

Plant Points
6.5

Naked fruit crumble

Serves **4**   Prep **10 mins**   Cook **30–40 mins (depending on the fruit)**

 Zero waste

This comforting dessert brings back memories of digging into my granny's fruit crumble. I pop this in the oven as I sit down to dinner; by the time I'm finished, the baked fruit, nut and cinnamon aromas have filled the kitchen and it's ready to eat. This recipe works all year round with whatever fruit is in season, and contains double the fibre (not to mention the plant diversity) of a lone piece of fruit.

4 large extra ripe nectarines, peaches, apples or pears, or a mix of each (approx. 600g)
6 Medjool dates, made into a paste (see page 134), or 6 tbsp sweetener of choice
1 tbsp extra virgin olive oil
40g mixed nuts, chopped
40g whole oats
½ tsp ground cinnamon
juice of 1 lemon (approx. 45ml), plus zest to taste

Topper:
50g live thick yoghurt, or cream-less ice cream (page 277)

Preheat the oven to *190°C/170°C fan/gas mark 5*.

Cut your fruit in half (if there is a core, remove it) and make a small hollow the size of a 50p coin. If using stone fruit, simply remove the stone.

Place the fruit in a small roasting tin, cut side up. You want the fruit to sit snugly inside the tin, so they don't dry out. Set aside.

Mix the date paste, olive oil and 1 tbsp of water together in a bowl, then add the nuts, oats, cinnamon and lemon juice. Mix until you have a sticky crumble mixture. Taste and adjust zest to preference.

Fill the hollows of the fruit with even amounts of the crumble.

Cover with foil and bake in the oven for 20 minutes (or 30 minutes if using apples or pears), then remove the foil and bake for a further 10–15 minutes until the crumble is golden brown and the fruit is tender.

Serve with your choice of yoghurt or ice cream.

Tip Short on time? Cook the fruit in the microwave for a few minutes first to soften it (approx. 3–4 minutes), before adding the crumble and baking for 10 minutes uncovered in the oven, or until golden brown.

Storage Best served straight out of the oven. Keeps in the fridge for up to 3 days.

Switch Already had oats this week? Switch them for rye flakes.

Gut-loving carrot cake with vanilla cream frosting

Serves **12**   Prep **25 mins, plus chilling**

 Zero waste

This plant-packed cake is my raw and vegan version of a classic carrot cake – perfectly sweet, rich and indulgent, it also nourishes your gut microbes. With each slice offering almost 6g of fibre, it's the perfect crowd-pleasing dessert to share with your foodie friends, and there are two toppers to choose from depending on how much time you have on your hands.

18 Medjool dates, pitted and roughly chopped (approx. 300g)
1½ tsp ground cinnamon
½ tsp ground ginger
¼ tsp nutmeg powder
3 medium carrots, grated (approx. 250g)
200g walnuts
100g pecans
100g ground almonds
60g raisins

Toppers:
250ml plant-based double cream (look for one that says 'for whipping')
1 tsp vanilla extract
10 walnuts, crumbled

or

350g cashews
250ml coconut cream
1 tsp vanilla extract
60ml honey
juice of ½ lemon (approx. 25ml), plus zest to taste

Storage Keeps in the fridge, in an airtight container, for 5 days.

Tip If you have any cake mixture left over, it's great for rolling into raw carrot cake snack balls!

Line a high-sided 20cm cake tin with non-stick baking paper on the base and sides, and set aside.

Blitz the dates with the spices (cinnamon, ginger and nutmeg) in a food processor for a minute or two, until it makes a ball. Add the carrot and pulse to combine roughly, then transfer to a mixing bowl.

Blitz the walnuts and pecans in the food processor until they form slightly chunky crumbs (approx. 20 seconds), then add to the mixing bowl along with the ground almonds and raisins. Use a wooden spoon to combine everything.

Tip the mix into the lined tin and press down to compress and smooth the top. Leave in the fridge to chill until you're ready to make the topping.

When you're ready to eat, whip the cream with the vanilla extract until it makes soft peaks. Spoon the cream on to the cake, sprinkle with the crumbled walnuts and serve.

For the alternative, more luxurious topping, cover the cashews with boiling water and set aside to soak for at least 10 minutes while you make the cake. Strain the soaked cashews and tip them into a high-powered food processor along with the other topper ingredients. Blitz on a high speed for 5–6 minutes until super-smooth, scraping down the sides occasionally. Pour over the carrot cake base and smooth out the top. Place in the fridge to set for around 4 hours.

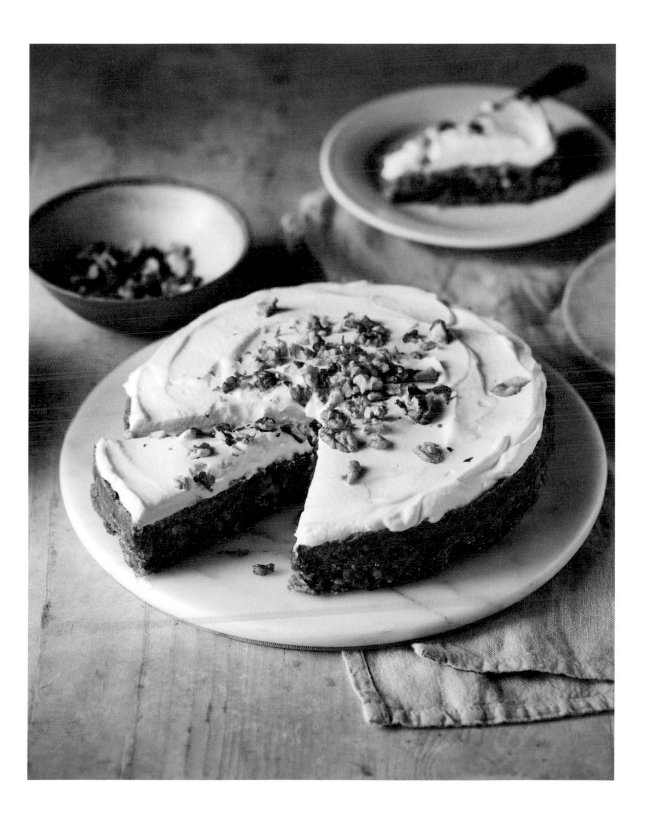

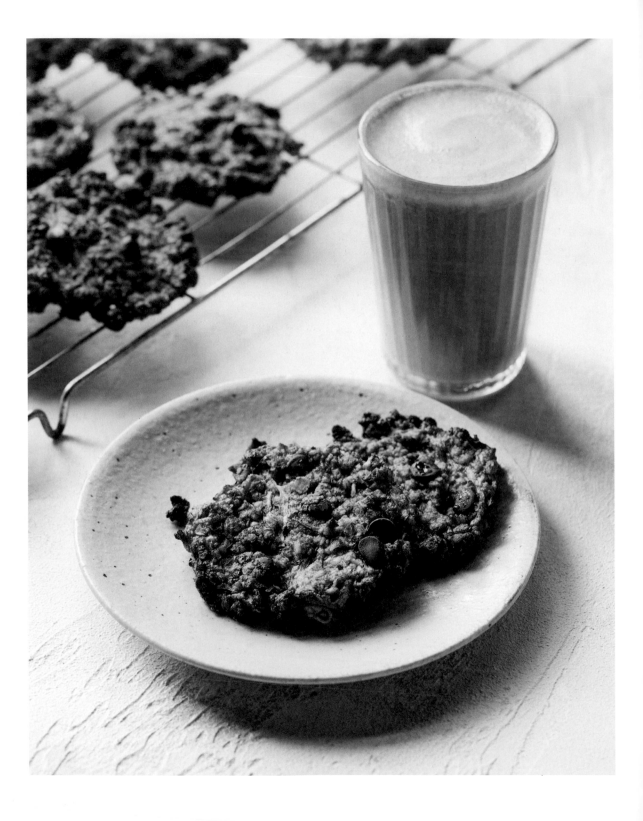

Choc chip courgette cookies

Plant Points
4.5

Makes **18 cookies**   Prep **15 mins**   Cook **25 mins**

 FODMAP Lite   **Freezer**   **Zero waste**

My answer to those biscuit barrel cravings. Combining the best of both worlds, these high-fibre choc chip cookies are a little crunchy and a little chewy, just like a good cookie should be. Plus, the hidden veg gives you an extra 4 plant points in one – and the kids will never know!

1 very ripe banana (approx. 100g)

6 Medjool dates, pitted and roughly chopped (approx. 100g)

50ml extra virgin olive oil

2 tsp vanilla extract

1 courgette, grated (approx. 140g prepped)

60g dark chocolate chips, or chocolate chips of choice

150g whole oats

Preheat the oven to *190°C/160°C/gas mark 4* and grease two baking trays with olive oil.

Place the banana and dates in a food processor along with the olive oil, half the oats and vanilla, and blitz for approx. 1 minute, until you have a paste.

Squeeze the grated courgette in a clean cloth to remove the excess moisture, before placing in a mixing bowl, along with the chocolate chips, remaining whole oats and the contents of the food processor. Stir well to combine into a thick mix.

Spoon the mix on to the baking trays, making approx. 18 cookies, and gently smooth into flat rounds.

Place in the oven and bake for 25–30 minutes until golden brown on the outside. Transfer to a wire rack and leave to cool completely.

Storage Best eaten fresh from the rack. Can be frozen baked or as raw dough for up to 1 month.

Drinks

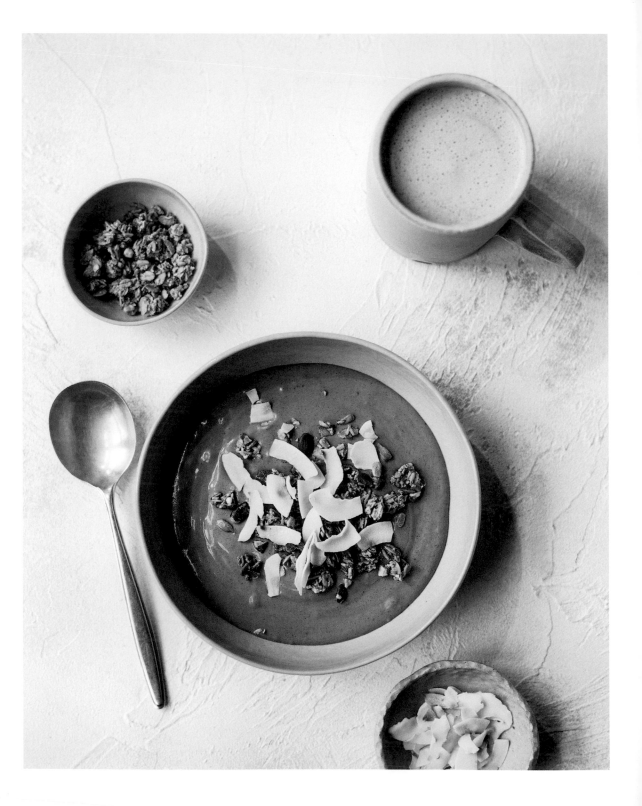

Snickers smoothie bowl

Serves **1 hungry person**   Prep **5 mins, plus freezing**

 Freezer

Move over ultra-processed protein shakes, this bowl not only offers 18g of protein, 10g of fibre and 6.25 plant points, but it tastes just like a Snickers chocolate bar – without the added sugar and additives.

60g silken tofu
50g live thick yoghurt
1 tbsp unsweetened cocoa powder
1 frozen very ripe banana (approx. 100g)
1 tbsp nut butter of choice
40g courgette, frozen
2 Medjool dates, pitted (approx. 30g)

Toppers (optional):
5g coconut flakes
16g granola (see page 143 for my
   no-added-sugar version)

Blitz the smoothie ingredients in a high-powered blender for approx. 1 minute, until smooth – layering in the frozen ingredients first for a smooth blend.

Pour into a small bowl or glass cup and add your choice of toppers.

Switch After a lighter option? Blitz in 70g of ice with a little extra water to thin, and share with a friend. Alternatively, freeze the leftovers in an ice cube tray, and when you're ready for round two, blitz together the frozen cubes and a little milk of choice. Keeps in the freezer for up to 1 month.

Tip If you add the granola from page 143, you'll get an extra 18.5 plant points.

Smoothies – Four Ways

Brain-boosting blueberry smoothie

Serves **1**   Prep **5 mins**

 Zero waste

Packed full of flavonoids shown to have brain-boosting properties, plus extra plant points and live microbes for good measure, this celebrates all the good that plants can do for our brain power.

100g frozen blueberries
1 ripe pear, chopped (approx. 110g)
2 florets frozen cauliflower (approx. 60g) (optional)
100g live thick yoghurt
100ml water, or milk of choice
ice, to serve

Place all the ingredients in a high-powered blender and blitz until smooth (layer in the frozen ingredients first for a smooth blend). Serve over ice and enjoy.

Switch Want to up your plant points? Switch the blueberries for mixed berries.

Immunity-nourishing smoothie

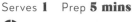

Serves **1**   Prep **5 mins**

 FODMAP Lite

Feeding your immune system while also satisfying your taste buds, this one is a bit of a no-brainer (remember 70 per cent of your immune cells live in your gut!). This is my go-to combo when winter season strikes, but also when I'm craving something refreshing on a hot summer's day. This beauty serves up 10g of fibre – that's a third of your daily intake in one glass.

1 large orange, peeled and halved (approx. 200g)
1 carrot, halved (approx. 70g)
½ very ripe banana (approx. 50g)
15g fresh ginger, peeled
20g walnuts
7 cubes of ice (approx. 100g)
80ml soy milk, or milk of choice
a big pinch of turmeric

Place all the ingredients in a high-powered blender and blitz for 1 minute or until smooth (add the ice first for a smooth blend). Taste and adjust ginger, turmeric and banana (for sweetness) to your preference.

Switch Had enough of carrots? Switch for 70g courgette.

Greenie crush

Plant Points
4.25

Serves **1**　Prep **5 mins**

Creamy and refreshing, plus it's packing 7g of fibre and 4 plant points per smoothie, your gut will thank you for making the switch from your fibre-stripped green juice.

1 apple, roughly chopped (approx. 150g)
½ cucumber, roughly chopped (approx. 70g)
¼ avocado (approx. 40g flesh)
50g silken tofu
7 mint leaves, more to taste
5 cubes of ice (approx. 70g)
80ml milk of choice

Place all the ingredients in a high-powered blender, and blitz for 1 minute or until smooth (add in the ice first for a smooth blend). Taste and adjust the mint to your preference, and add additional plant milk/water/ice to achieve your preferred thickness.

Switch No mint? Switch for 10g fresh ginger.

Raspberry red

Plant Points
6

Serves **1**　Prep **5 mins**

Forget those sickly sweet fruit-only smoothies – this combo is not only satisfyingly creamy but offers plenty of plant-based diversity. A winning breakfast, snack or post-workout fuel, it has over 10g of fibre and 15g of protein per portion.

80g frozen raspberries
1 celery stick (approx. 50g)
20g porridge oats
20g dried cranberries, or sweetener of choice
1 tbsp almond butter
80g live thick yoghurt
5 cubes of ice (approx. 70g)
20g raw beetroot (optional)

Place all the ingredients in a high-powered blender along with 80ml water and blitz for 1–2 minutes or until smooth (add in the ice first for a smooth blend). Taste and adjust flavours to preference. Best served over ice.

Switch Love kefir? Me too! Swap the yoghurt and water for 150ml of kefir.

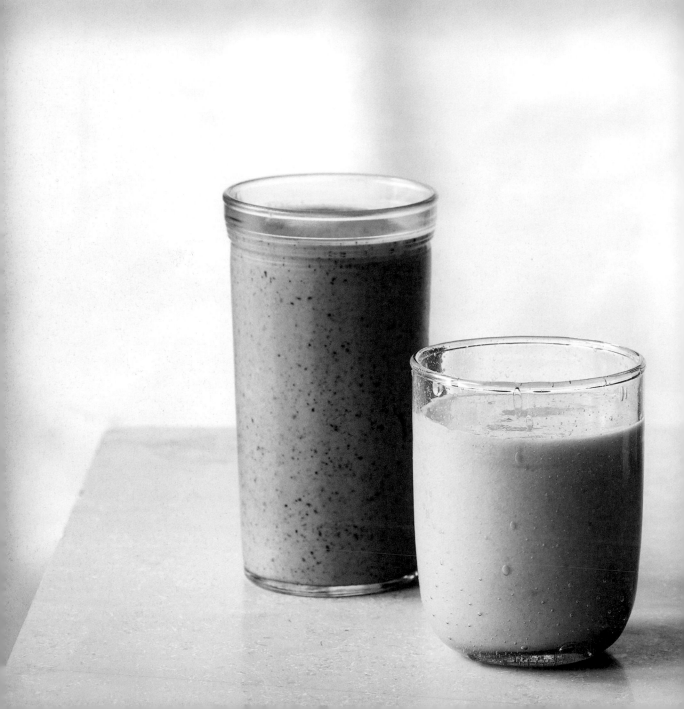

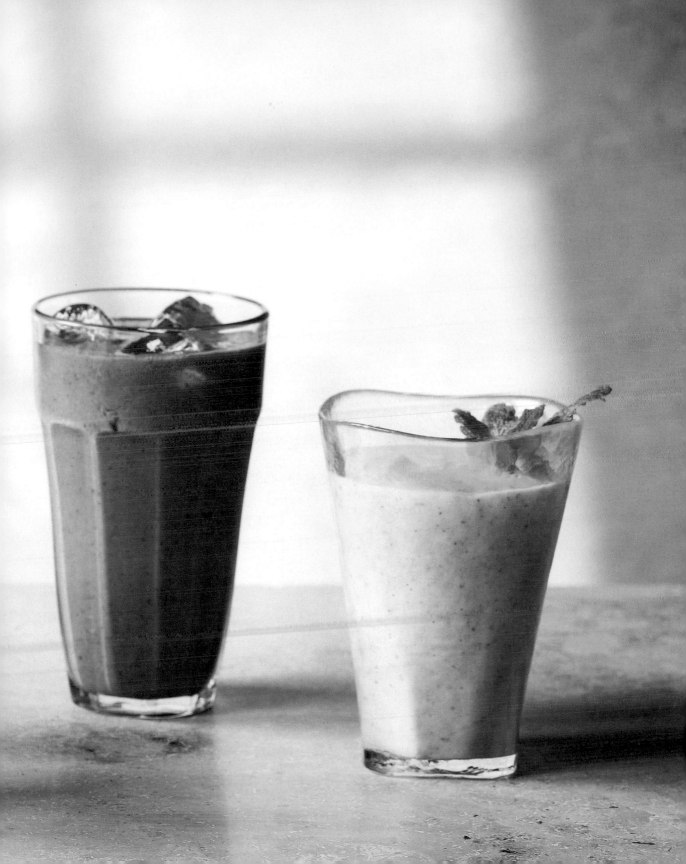

Microbe-made ginger soda

Plant Points
0.25

Makes **8 x 240ml servings**   Prep **3 weeks (approx. 4–7 days for ginger bug; 10–14 days for ginger soda)**

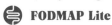 **FODMAP Lite**

Before machines, all sparkling drinks were microbe-made, so here's to bringing back the good old ways for a homemade refreshing fizz. If you want to experiment with the microbial world, but aren't quite ready for kefir or kombucha, then this is the recipe for you.

Step 1: Ginger bug

2 tsp fresh ginger, grated skin and all, per day
2 tsp white sugar, per day
250ml filtered water

Equipment:
500ml glass jar, sterilized
clean cloth
elastic band

Add 2 tsp ginger, 2 tsp sugar and 250ml filtered water to the glass jar. Stir to dissolve the sugar, and cover with the cloth and elastic band.

Each day for the next 4–7 days, stir in an additional 2 tsp of ginger and 2 tsp of sugar (think of this as feeding the community of microbes). Give the jar a little swirl whenever you walk past it (aim for at least twice per day), as this helps evenly distribute the food to the microbes.

Depending on the climate (faster in summer, longer in winter), by day 4 bubbles should start to appear in the jar (this is a sign the microbes are busy eating the sugar). Once the ginger has floated to the top of the jar and there are bubbles on the surface, your ginger bug is ready for graduation – you can move on to step 2.

Tip If there are no bubbles by day 7, it's best to ditch the batch and start again (there may not have been enough microbes in and on your ginger – try using organic ginger for the next batch if you haven't already).

Step 2: Ginger soda

1.75 litres water (tap is fine, as you'll boil this)

175g white or brown sugar (don't worry, you won't be consuming all of this)

2–4 tbsp fresh ginger, grated, to taste

250ml strained ginger bug (from step 1)

juice of 1 lemon (approx. 50ml)

Equipment:

2 x 1-litre airtight sterilized glass bottles

In a large saucepan, boil the water, ginger and sugar for around 10 minutes with the lid on. Taste the mix and adjust the ginger to preferred flavour intensity. It will taste rather sweet, but rest assured the microbes from your ginger bug will eat a lot of this sugar over the next 2 weeks.

Once completely cool, add in the ginger bug and lemon juice and stir to combine. Decant the mix into the two bottles, being sure to leave some headspace for the bubbles that the ginger bug will produce.

Seal the lids and leave to ferment in a dark cupboard at room temperature for around 2 weeks (ideally between 18°C and 24°C). Like the ginger bug, the warmer the tempeature the faster the microbes work, so be sure to adjust how long you leave it by the time of year. Every third day, open the lid to release the pressure and give it a little taste. You should notice the bubbles increasing over time as the sweetness settles.

Once it hits your preferred level of carbonation and sweetness, place it in the fridge (this will put the microbes to sleep) and, once chilled, enjoy a refreshing bubbly cup!

Storage Best consumed within 2 weeks, although I doubt it'll lust that long.

Frothy cashew latte

Plant Points
2.25

Serves **1**   Prep **5 mins**

 FODMAP Lite   **Zero waste**

Forget all the soaking and straining faff, this nutty latte uses whole cashews, saving you time and giving you an extra hit of gut-loving prebiotic fibre. Did I mention it's deliciously creamy too? A must-try!

1 cup of hot coffee (approx. 250ml), made to your strength preference
30g roasted cashew nuts
1 Medjool date

Place all the ingredients in a high-powered blender and blitz for 1 minute or until smooth. Taste and adjust flavours to preference.

Tip For extra indulgence, use salted roasted cashews for a flavour explosion! And while, yes, they contain a little added salt, in the grand scheme of the Diversity Diet that's rather negligible.

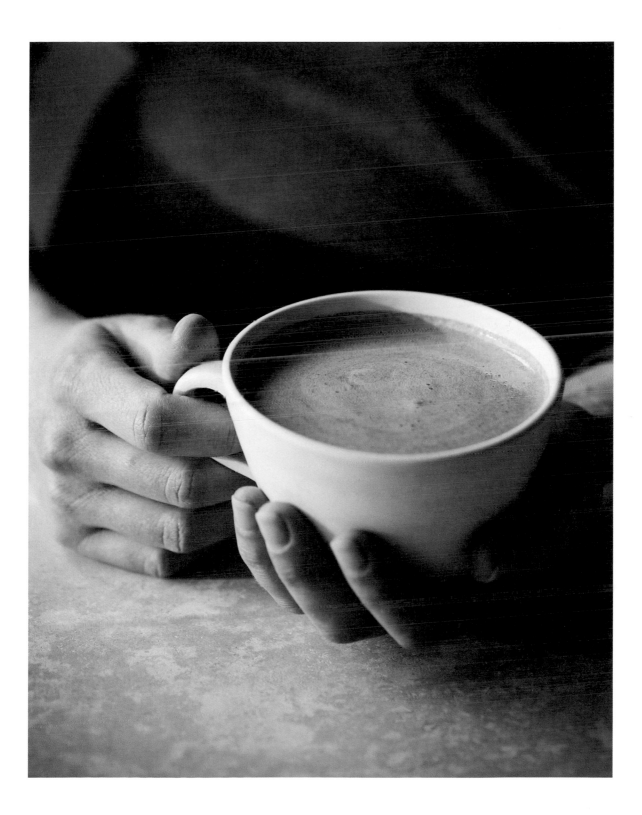

One-minute snacks

Sweet potato slider: Leftover cooked sweet potato with nut butter and a dollop of live yoghurt.

🌀 **FODMAP Lite**

Prebiotic 'chocolate' milkshake: Add 250ml of your milk of choice, 1 tbsp cocoa, 1 tbsp nut butter of choice, ¼ tsp vanilla extract and 2 Medjool dates to a high-powered blender, and blitz.

🌀 **FODMAP Lite**

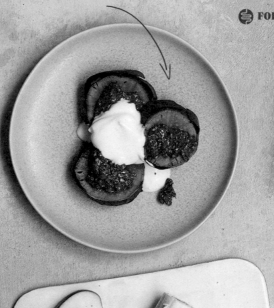

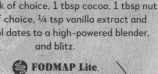

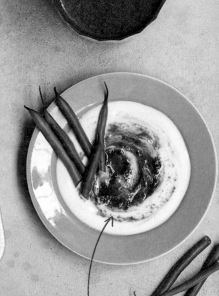

Apple slider: Apple, pecans and cinnamon.

🌀 **FODMAP Lite**

Banana bites: Banana circles glued together with nut butter and desiccated coconut.

🌀 **FODMAP Lite**

Bean dippers: Live yoghurt with a teaspoon of harissa paste or wholegrain mustard stirred through, served with raw green beans or sugar snap peas.

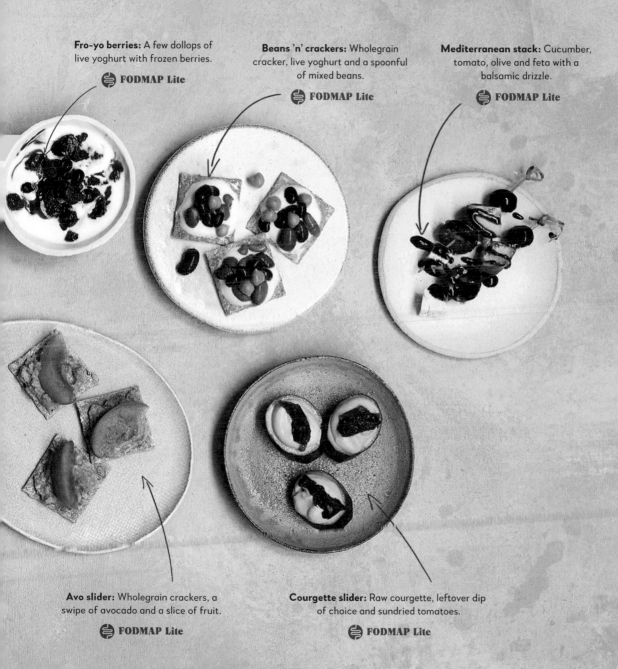

Fro-yo berries: A few dollops of live yoghurt with frozen berries.

FODMAP Lite

Beans 'n' crackers: Wholegrain cracker, live yoghurt and a spoonful of mixed beans.

FODMAP Lite

Mediterranean stack: Cucumber, tomato, olive and feta with a balsamic drizzle.

FODMAP Lite

Avo slider: Wholegrain crackers, a swipe of avocado and a slice of fruit.

FODMAP Lite

Courgette slider: Raw courgette, leftover dip of choice and sundried tomatoes.

FODMAP Lite

FODMAP-lite recipe switches

	Recipe	Portion size/switch
Breakfast	Muffin in a mug (page 138)	Stick to one portion and switch out dates for maple syrup.
	Omelette bowl (page 139)	Use dried chives instead of onion granules, and use tinned peas (rinsed well).
	Fibre-filled breakfast wrap (page 141)	Ensure tofu is firm (not silken); reduce avocado portion to 30g; switch out wholemeal wrap for gluten-free variety.
	No-bake bites (page 142)	Stick to a portion of 1–2 balls.
	DIY plant-packed muesli (page 143)	Opt for rice, corn or quinoa flakes. Switch out dried mango and apple for dried cranberries/raisins/sultanas or freeze-dried berries. Stick to a 50g portion.
	Crispy bacon-shrooms with creamy butter bean hummus (page 144)	Switch out portobello mushrooms for oyster mushrooms, and dates for maple syrup. Spread the hummus thinly; instead of garlic and olive oil opt for garlic-infused oil. Stick to one slice of sourdough or switch out for a gluten-free option.
	Mango and berry fro-yo slice (page 146)	Stick to half a portion, and eat with additional live yoghurt or FODMAP-lite muesli on the side (see DIY plant-packed muesli, page 143).
	Plant-powered baked oat slice (page 148)	Stick to 1 portion. Opt for almond milk, and switch out dates for maple syrup.
	Breakfast pitta pizza (page 151)	Switch out pitta bread for a gluten-free pitta/wrap. Use only the green parts of the spring onion, and ensure the sundried tomatoes don't include garlic or onion. Use half a portion of the base sauce and stick to 30g of avocado.
	Eat-the-rainbow pancake stack (page 153)	Stick to 2 small pancakes, topped with live yoghurt and maple syrup.
Sweet treats	Loaded melon wedges (page 157)	Switch out watermelon for honeydew melon, and stick to 80g. For the berry whip option: switch out blackberries for blueberries, and honey for maple syrup. If using choc hazelnut spread, keep to a 2 tbsp portion.
	Ultimate raspberry and white choc muffins (page 161)	Switch out wholemeal flour for gluten-free flour, and dates for maple syrup.

	Recipe	Portion size/switch
Light bites	Garlicky aquafaba aioli (page 170)	Switch out garlic for 1 tbsp of garlic-infused olive oil.
	Smoky aubergine dip (page 172)	Switch out garlic and olive oil for garlic-infused olive oil.
	No-added-sugar ketchup (page 173)	Stick to a 2 tbsp portion and reduce onion to 50g. Switch out dates for maple syrup.
	Seedy cracker duo (page 175)	Switch out rye flour for gluten-free flour.
	Snack-o-clock veg fritters (page 179)	Switch out wholemeal flour for gluten-free flour, and use veg options from page 309.
	All-the-greens filo swirl (page 180)	Stick to one serving. Use tinned peas (rinsed well).
	Popcorn chick-less nuggets (page 183)	Switch out wholemeal flour for gluten-free flour.
	Butternut muffins (page 189)	Switch out spelt flour for gluten-free flour and butternut squash for sweet potato. Stick to maximum of 3 muffins per portion.
Packed lunches	Smoked mackerel, new potato and apple salad (page 195)	Switch out cashews for nut options (see page 309), and asparagus for green beans. Limit fennel to 180g, and switch out apples for 200g of grapes.
	Sweet jacket potato with black beans (page 196)	Switch out sweet potato for a regular potato, and garlic and olive oil for garlic-infused olive oil. Reduce black beans to 90g and add 150g of chopped tomatoes, peppers or veg (detailed on page 309). Limit avocado to 60g.
	Sweet jacket potato with nut-free pesto (page 197)	Switch out sweet potato for regular potato, and garlic and olive oil for garlic-infused olive oil. Limit butter beans to 90g and add 150g of chopped peppers or veg (detailed on page 309).
	PB & J sweet jacket potato (page 197)	Stick to half a sweet potato per portion (90g cooked) and opt for nut or seed butter (detailed on page 309).

	Recipe	Portion size/switch
Packed lunches	Chunky veg and feta frittata (page 201)	Replace red onion with the green part of a spring onion (80g).
	Tofu fried wholegrains with crunchy cashews (page 202)	Opt for a gluten-free wholegrain e.g. quinoa, buckwheat, wild rice. Switch out cashews for nuts and stir-fry veg for other veg options (see list on page 309). Use only the green part of the spring onion (10g) and tinned peas (rinsed well). Switch out silken tofu for firm (or opt for an egg), and garlic for 1 tbsp of garlic-infused olive oil.
	Reinvented chicken burger (page 205)	Use a gluten-free bun.
	Thai-inspired fishcakes and crunchy salad (page 210)	Use only the green part of the spring onion.
Weeknight dinners	Stir-fry adventures	Protein: If using tinned beans, limit to 45g per serving and add additional firm tofu, peanuts, eggs, fish or lean meat Wholegrains: Opt for gluten-free wholegrains (see page 309 for options). Veg: See page 309 for options.
	Stir fry – Indian (page 216)	Switch out garlic and olive oil for garlic-infused olive oil, and cauliflower for any suggested veg on page 309.
	Stir fry – Italian (page 217)	Switch out garlic and olive oil for garlic-infused olive oil.
	Stir fry – Korean (page 217)	Opt for gochujang paste, or go without if sensitive to chilli.
	Stir fry – Indonesian (page 218)	Switch out shallots for the green part of a spring onion.
	Stir fry – Thai (page 218)	Switch out the garlic and olive oil for garlic-infused olive oil, and the mangetout or sugar snap peas for pak choi or fine green beans. Use only the green part of the spring onion.
	Orange-glazed roasted salmon (page 226)	Switch out the garlic for ½ tbsp of garlic-infused olive oil, and the date paste for maple syrup. Serve with gluten-free wholegrains (see options on page 309). Use only the green part of the spring onion.
	Easy noodle broth (page 229)	Use onion- and garlic-free vegetable stock, and soba (buckwheat) or rice noodles. Opt for firm tofu rather than silken. Use only the green part of the spring onion. Skip the chilli if sensitive.

	Recipe	Portion size/switch
Fancy dinners	Spinach and ricotta stuffed pasta shells (page 247)	Stick to half a portion, and switch out the garlic and olive oil for garlic-infused olive oil. Ensure the sundried tomatoes and passata don't include onion or garlic. Use gluten-free pasta shells, and tinned peas (rinsed well).
	Tear-and-share with butter bean relish (page 248)	Stick to half a portion and use a gluten-free loaf. Switch out the onion for 60g of the green part of spring onion, and dates for maple syrup.
	Chicken 'n' veg meaty balls (page 256)	Use gluten-free bread, and only the green part of the spring onion.
Sides	Greens and beans (page 263)	Switch out the garlic and olive oil for garlic-infused olive oil. Reduce beans to just one 400g tin. Stick to one portion.
	Sticky parsnips (page 264)	Use only the green part of the spring onion. Switch out garlic for 1 tbsp of garlic-infused olive oil, and date paste for maple syrup. Use gluten-free flour.
	Veg all-dressed-up (page 265)	Only use the avocado pesto (creamy cashew not appropriate). Switch out the garlic and olive oil for garlic-infused olive oil. Opt for gluten-free wraps.
	Spinach balls with tahini sauce (page 268)	Switch out date paste for maple syrup.
	Quinoa rice with hoisin drizzle (page 271)	Switch out the garlic for 1 tsp of garlic-infused olive oil, and date paste for maple syrup. Use only the green part of the spring onions. Skip the chilli if sensitive.
Desserts	Raspberry and lemon ricotta baked cheesecake (page 275)	Switch out the honey for maple syrup.
	Trail mix loaf cake with yoghurt and white chocolate glaze (page 276)	Stick to 1 portion. Use gluten-free flour, and switch out the dried mango and figs for cranberries/raisins/sultanas/goji berries.
	Cream-less ice cream – two ways (page 277–8)	Hidden veg: Stick to half a portion, switch out dates for maple syrup, and opt for choc mint as filling option. No freeze: Stick to 1 portion. Use blueberries, raspberries or strawberries.
	Prebiotic rocky road (page 281)	Stick to 1 portion. Replace the dried mango and figs with 120g of dried banana chips.
	Prebiotic pistachio berry bursts (page 282)	Stick to 2 or 3 per portion.
	Choc chip courgette cookies (page 289)	Switch out the Medjool dates for maple syrup.

	Recipe	Portion size/switch
Drinks	Immunity-nourishing smoothie (page 294)	Reduce the orange to 100g and add 1 tsp of maple syrup. Switch out the soy milk for almond milk.
	Frothy cashew latte (page 300)	Switch out the cashews for peanuts, and the date for maple syrup. If you are sensitive to caffeine, switch to decaf coffee.
One-minute snacks (pages 302–303)	Sweet potato slider	Keep to 80g of sweet potato, and switch out nut and seed butters (see page 309).
	Prebiotic 'chocolate' milkshake	Opt for cow's or almond milk, nut and seed butters from page 309, and switch out dates for maple syrup.
	Fro-yo berries	Keep to a maximum of 80g of berries, and choose between blueberries, cranberries, raspberries and strawberries.
	Courgette slider	Ensure dip doesn't contain onion or garlic.
	Apple slider	Switch out apple for 60g of banana, honeydew melon or fruit options (see page 309).
	Banana bites	Stick to 60g of banana, and opt for nut and seed butters from page 309.
	Avo slider	Keep to 2 crackers, 30g of avocado and 80g of fruit options listed on page 309.
	Beans 'n' crackers	Keep to 2 crackers and 45g of tinned mixed beans (triple-rinsed).

Select higher-FODMAP foods to limit	Examples of alternatives*
Veg Artichokes, asparagus, broccoli, Brussels sprouts, cabbage, cauliflower, chicory root, garlic, leeks, mushrooms, onions, peas, spring onions (white part).	Aubergines, carrots, chives, courgettes, cucumber, ginger, green beans, kale, peppers, pickled garlic and onion, potatoes, pumpkin, spinach, tomatoes.
Fruit Apples, apricots, blackberries, boysenberries, cherries, dates, figs, mango, nectarines, peaches, pears, persimmons (Sharon fruit), plums, prunes, watermelon, fruit juice (more than 100ml), foods/drinks with added fruit concentrate.	Blueberries, clementines, grapes, honeydew melon, kiwis, lemons, limes, oranges, passion fruit, pineapple, raspberries, rhubarb, strawberries. Maximum of 1 piece of any fruit per sitting (equivalent of 80g fresh, 30g dried, 100ml juice), with a maximum of three sittings across the day.
Protein sources Legumes (e.g. baked beans, chickpeas, kidney beans, soya beans), pistachio nuts and cashews.	All fresh meats (e.g. chicken, fish, lamb), eggs, firm tofu, walnuts, Brazil nuts. Peanuts, sunflower or pumpkin seeds, whole or as nut/seed butters. Tinned and (thoroughly) rinsed legumes, contain fewer FODMAPs compared to those boiled from dry. Therefore, small portions (¼ cup per sitting), particularly of tinned chickpeas, butter beans and adzuki beans, are better tolerated. ½ cup of tinned lentils is considered low-FODMAP.
Wholegrains Keep to ½ cup of cooked or 1 slice of wheat, barley or rye-based foods per sitting (including couscous and semolina), with up to three across the day.	Quinoa, rice, buckwheat, millet, oats, polenta.
Other Agave, honey, high-fructose corn syrup, fructose and low-calorie sweeteners ending in -ol (see page 143 of *Eat Yourself Healthy*). Added inulin, fructo-oligosaccharide, galacto-oligosaccharide in some yoghurts and cereals.	Golden syrup, maple syrup, table sugar (sucrose), glucose.

*This is not a comprehensive list, instead it is to give you inspiration. Include all other foods that are not listed on the 'higher-FODMAP' column in your diet. Remember this is a modified version, not the full low-FODMAP diet.

References

Introduction: Plant-based eating – redefined

Evelyn Medawar et al., 'The Effects of Plant-Based Diets on the Body and the Brain: A Systematic Review', *Translational Psychiatry*, vol. 9, article 226, September 2019.

https://www.vegansociety.com/news/media/statistics.

Chapter 1: So what *is* plant-based eating, exactly?

Mark L. Heiman and Frank L. Greenway, 'A Healthy Gastrointestinal Microbiome Is Dependent on Dietary Diversity', *Molecular Metabolism*, vol. 5, no. 5, May 2016, pp. 317–320, https://doi.org/10.1016/j.molmet.2016.02.005.

https://www.thelancet.com/article/SO140-6376(18)31809-9/fulltext

Laura E. Martin, Kristen E. Kay and Ann-Marie Torregrossa, 'Bitter-Induced Salivary Proteins Increase Detection Threshold of Quinine, But Not Sucrose', *Chemical Senses*, vol. 44, no. 6, July 2019, pp. 379–388, https://doi.org/10.1093/chemse/bjz021.

J. Poore and T. Nemecek, 'Reducing Food's Environmental Impacts Through Producers and Consumers', *Science*, vol. 360, no. 6392, June 2018, pp. 987–992, https://doi.org/10.1126/science.aaq0216.

Peter Scarborough et al., 'Dietary Greenhouse Gas Emissions of Meat-Eaters, Fish-Eaters, Vegetarians and Vegans in the UK', *Climatic Change*, vol. 125, 2014, pp. 179–192, https://link.springer.com/article/10.1007/s10584-014-1169-1.

Walter Willett et al., 'Food in the Anthropocene: The EAT-Lancet Commission on Healthy Diets from Sustainable Food Systems', *The Lancet*, vol. 393, no. 10170, February 2019, pp. 447–492, https://pubmed.ncbi.nlm.nih.gov/30660336/.

L. A. Wyness et al., 'Reducing the Population's Sodium Intake: The UK Food Standard Agency's Salt Reduction Programme', *Public Health Nutrition*, vol. 15, no. 2, February 2012, pp. 254–261, https://doi.org/10.1017.S1368980011000966.

Chapter 2: What are plant-based foods?

Francisco Asnicar and Sarah E. Berry, 'Microbiome Connections with Host Metabolism and Habitual Diet from 1,098 Deeply Phenotyped Individuals', *Nature Medicine*, vol. 27, 2021, pp. 331–332, https://doi.org/10.1038/s41591-020-01183-8.

Gabriele Berg et al., 'Microbiome Definition Re-visited: Old Concepts and New Challenges', *Microbiome*, vol. 8, article 103, 2020, https://microbiomejournal.biomedcentral.com/articles/10.1186/s40168-020-00875-0.

Jeanelle Boyer and Rui Hai Liu, 'Apple Phytochemicals and Their Health Benefits', *Nutrition Journal*, vol. 3, article 5, 2004, https://doi.org/10.1186/1475-2891-3-5.

Matteo Briguglio et al., 'Dietary Neurotransmitters: A Narrative Review on Current Knowledge', *Nutrients*, vol. 10, no. 5, May 2018, p591, https://doi.org/10.3390/nu10050591.16

British Nutrition Foundation, 'Protein', https://www.nutrition.org.uk/nutritionscience/nutrients-food-and-ingredients/protein.

R. Deewatthanawong and C. B. Watkins, 'Accumulation of γ-Aminobutyric Acid in Apple, Strawberry and Tomato Fruit in Response to Postharvest Treatments', *Acta Horticulturae*, vol. 877: VI International Postharvest Symposium, April 2009, https://www.researchgate.net/publication/248381932_Accumulation_of_g-Aminobutyric_Acid_in_Apple_Strawberry_and_Tomato_Fruit_in_Response_to_Postharvest_Treatments.

Emmanuelle Dheilly et al., 'Cell Wall Dynamics During Apple Development and Storage Involves Hemicellulose Modifications and Related Expressed Genes', *BMC Plant Biology*, vol. 6, article 201, 2016, https://doi.org/10.1186/s12870-016-0887-0.

Yan Hou et al., 'Anti-Depressant Natural Flavanols Modulate BDNF and Beta Amyloid in Neurons and Hippocampus of Double TgAD Mice', *Neuropharmacology*, vol. 58, no. 6, May 2010, pp. 911–920, https://doi.org/10.1016/j.neuropharm.2009.11.002.

Francisco Javier-Ruiz-Ojeda et al., 'Effects of Sweeteners on the Gut Microbiota: A Review of Experimental Studies and Clinical Trials', *Advances in Nutrition*, vol. 10, supplement 1, January 2019, pp. S31–S48, https://doi.org/10.1093/advances/nmy037.

Abigail J. Johnson et al., 'Daily Sampling Reveals Personalized Diet-Microbiome Associations in Humans', *Cell Host & Microbe*, vol. 25, no. 6, June 2019, pp. 789–802.e5, https://doi.org/10.1016/j.chom.2019.05.005

Mark L. Heiman and Frank L. Greenway, 'A Healthy Gastrointestinal Microbiome Is Dependent on Dietary Diversity', *Molecular Metabolism*, vol. 5, no. 5, May 2016, pp. 317–320, https://doi.org/10.1016/j.molmet.2016.02.005.

V. Juturu, J. P. Bowman and J. Deshpande, 'Overall Skin Tone and Skin-Lightening-Improving Effects with Oral Supplementation of Lutein and Zeaxanthin Isomers: A Double-Blind, Placebo-Controlled Clinical Trial', *Clinical, Cosmetic and Investigational Dermatology*, vol. 9, 2016, pp. 325–332, https://doi.org/10.2147/CCID.S115519.

Josephine Kschonsek et al., 'Polyphenolic Compounds Analysis of Old and New Apple Cultivars and Contribution of Polyphenolic Profile to the In Vitro Antioxidant Capacity', *Antioxidants*, vol. 71, no. 1, January 2018, p. 20, https://doi.org/10.3390/antiox7010020.

François Mariotti and Christopher D. Gardner, 'Dietary Protein and Amino Acids in Vegetarian Diets – A Review', *Nutrients*, vol. 11, no. 1, November 2019, p. 2661, https://doi.org/10.3390/nu11112661.

Carlos Augusto Monteiro at al., 'Household Availability of Ultra-Processed Foods and Obesity in Nineteen European Countries', *Public Health Nutrition*, vol. 21, Special Issue 1: *Ultra Processed Foods*, January 2018, pp. 8–26, https://doi.org/10.1017/S1368980017001379.

Leonardo Nogueira, 'Epicatechin Enhances Fatigue Resistance and Oxidative Capacity in Mouse Muscle', *Journal of Physiology*, vol. 589, no. 18, September 2011, pp. 4615–4631, https://doi.org/10.1113/jphysiol.2011.209924.

M. Poyet et al., 'A Library of Human Gut Bacterial Isolates Paired with Longitudinal Multiomics Data Enables Mechanistic Microbiome Research', *Nature Medicine*, vol. 24, September 2019, pp. 1442–1452, https://www.nature.com/articles/s41591-019-0559-3

Marion Salomé et al., 'Plant-Protein Diversity Is Critical to Ensuring the Nutritional Adequacy of Diets When Replacing Animal with Plant Protein: Observed and Modeled Diets of French Adults', *Journal of Nutrition*, vol. 50, no. 3, March 2020, pp. 536–545, https://doi.org/10.1093/jn/nxz252.

Ambika Satya et al., 'Healthful and Unhealthful Plant-Based Diets and the Risk of Coronary Heart Disease in US Adults', *Journal of the American College of Cardiology*, vol. 70, no. 4, July 2017, pp. 411–422, https://doi.org/10.1016/j.jacc.2017.05.047.

Bruno Senghor et al., 'Gut Microbiota Diversity According to Dietary Habits and Geographical Provenance', *Human Microbiome Journal*, vols 7–8, April 2018, pp. 1–9, https://doi.org/10.1016/j.humic.2018.01.001.

E. Thom, 'The Effect of Chlorogenic Acid Enriched Coffee on Glucose Absorption in Healthy Volunteers and Its Effect on Body Mass When Used Long-Term in Overweight and Obese People', *Journal of International Medical Research*, vol. 35, no. 6, November 2007, pp. 900–908, https://doi.org/10.1177/147323000703500620.

Birgit Wassermann, Henry Müller and Gabriele Berg, 'An Apple a Day: Which Bacteria Do We Eat with Organic and Conventional Apples?', *Frontiers in Microbiology*, 24 July 2019, https://doi.org/10.3389/fmicb.2019.01620.

Anna Wojciechowska et al., 'Insitols' Importance in the Improvement of the Endocrine–Metabolic Profile in PCOS', *International Journal of Molecular Sciences*, vol. 20, no. 22, November 2019, p. 5787, https://doi.org/10.3390/ijms20225787.

Haixia Zhang et al., 'Melatonin in Apples and Juice: Inhibition of Browning and Microorganism Growth in Apple Juice', *Molecules*, vol. 23, no. 3, February 2018, p. 521, https://doi.org/10.3390/molecules23030521.

Chapter 3: Why is going plant-based so important?

Anne Conolly and Sylvie Craig, *Health Survey for England 2018: Overweight and Obesity in Adults and Children*, NHS Digital, 3 December 2019, https://files.digital.nhs.uk/52/FD7E18/HSE18-Adult-Child-Obesity-rep.pdf.

Diabetes UK, 'Number of People Living with Diabetes Doubles in Twenty Years', 27 February 2018, https://www.diabetes.org.uk/about_us/news/diabetes-prevalence-statistics.

Food and Agriculture Organization of the United Nations, *The Second Report on the State of the World's Plant Genetic Resources for Food and Agriculture*, 2010, http://www.fao.org/3/i1500e/i1500e00.htm.

GBD 2017 Diet Collaborators, 'Health Effects of Dietary Risks in 195 Countries, 200–2017: A Systematic Analysis for the Global Burden of Disease Study 2017', *The Lancet*, vol. 393, no. 10184, May 2019, pp. 1958–1972, https://doi.org/10.1016/S0140-6736(19)30041-8.

Mark L. Heiman and Frank L. Greenway, 'A Healthy Gastrointestinal Microbiome Is Dependent on Healthy Diets from Sustainable Food Systems', *The Lancet*, vol. 393, no. 17170, February 2019, pp. 447–492, https://pubmed.ncbi.nlm.nih.gov/30660336/.

Susan J. Hewlings and Douglas S. Kalman, 'Curcumin: A Review of Its Effects on Human Health', *Foods*, vol. 6, no. 10, October 2017, p. 92, https://doi.org/10.3390/foods6100092.

Jonna Jalanka-Tuovinen et al., 'Intestinal Microbiota in Healthy Adults: Temporal Analysis Reveals Individual and Common Core and Relation to Intestinal Symptoms', *PloS One*, vol. 6, no. 7, 2011, e23035, https://doi.org/10.1371/journal.pone.0023035.

Natasha Khazai, Suzanne E. Judd and Vin Tangpricha, 'Calcium and Vitamin D: Skeletal and Extraskeletal Health', *Current Rheumatology Reports*, vol. 10, 2008, pp. 110–117, https://doi.org/10.1007/s11926-008-0020-y

C. M. Weaver, W. R. Proulx and R. Heaney, 'Choices for Achieving Adequate Dietary Calcium with a Vegetarian Diet', *American Journal of Clinical Nutrition*, vol. 70, no. 3, September 1999, pp. 543s–548s, https://doi.org/10.1093/ajcn/70.3.543s.

Andrew Kingston et al., 'Projections of Multi-Morbidity in the Older Population in England to 2035: Estimates from the Population Ageing and Care Simulation (PACSim) Model', *Age and Ageing* vol. 47, no. 3, May 2018, pp. 374–380, https://doi.org/10.1093/ageing/afx201.

Mental Health Foundation, 'Mental Health Statistics: UK and Worldwide', https://www.mentalhealth.org.uk/statistics/mental-health-statistics-uk-and-worldwide

Ravinder Nagpal et al., 'Gut Microbiome and Aging: Physiological and Mechanistic Insights', *Nutrition and Healthy Aging*, vol. 4, no. 4, June 2018, p. 267–285, https://doi.org/10.3233/NHA-170030.

S. M. K. Rates, 'Plants as Source of Drugs', *Toxicon*, vol. 39, no. 5, May 2001, pp. 603–613, https://doi.org/10.1016/S0041-0101(00)00154-9.

M. Rizwan et al., 'Tomato Paste Rich in Lycopene Protects Against Cutaneous Photodamage in Humans in Vivo: A Randomized Controlled Trial', *British Journal of Dermatology*, vol. 164, no. 1, January 2011, pp. 154–162, https://doi.org/10.1111/j.1365-2133.2010.10057.x.

Jan Philipp Schuchardt and Andreas Hahn, 'Intestinal Absorption and Factors Influencing Bioavailability of Magnesium', *Current Nutrition & Food Science*, vol. 13, no. 4, 2017, pp. 260–278, https://doi.org/10.2174/1573401313666170427162740.

Justin L. Sonnenburg and Erica D. Sonnenburg, 'Vulnerability of the Industrialized Microbiota', *Science*, vol. 366, no. 6464, 25 October 2019, https://doi.org/10.1126/science.aaw9255.

Chapter 4: The plant-based benefits

James M. Baker, Layla Al-Nakkash and Melissa M. Herbst-Kralovetz, 'Estrogen–Gut Microbiome Axis: Physiological and Clinical Implications', *Maturitas*, vol. 103, September 2017, pp. 45–53, https://doi.org/10.1016/j.maturitas.2017.06.025

Hui Zhao et al., 'Compositional and Functional Features of the Female Premenopausal and Postmenopausal Gut Microbiota', *FEBS Letters*, vol. 593, no. 18, July 2019, pp. 2655–2664, https://doi.org/10.1002/1873-3468.13527.

Tracey L. K. Bear et al., 'The Role of the Gut Microbiota in Dietary Interventions for Depression and Anxiety', *Advances in Nutrition*, vol. 11, no. 4, July 2020, pp. 890–907, https://doi.org/10.1093/advances/nmaa016.

Mauro Cozzolino et al., 'Therapy with Probiotics and Synbiotics for Polycystic Ovarian Syndrome: A Systematic Review and Meta-Analysis', *European Journal of Nutrition*, vol. 59, no. 7, May 2020, pp. 2841–2856, https://doi.org/10.1007.s00394-020-0223-0.

Gabriella d'Ettorre et al., 'Challenges in the Management of SARS-CoV-2 Infection: The Role of Oral Bacteriotherapy as Complementary Therapeutic Strategy to Avoid the Progression of COVID-19', *Frontiers in Medicine*, July 2020, https://doi.org/10.3389/fmed.2020.00389.

M. C. Flux and Christopher A. Lowry, 'Finding Intestinal Fortitude: Integrating the Microbiome into a Holistic View of Depression Mechanism, Treatment, and Resilience', *Neurobiology of Disease*, vol. 135, article 104578, February 2020, https://doi.org/10.1016/j.nbd.2019.104578.

Elizabeth A. Grice and Julia A. Segre, 'The Skin Microbiome', *Nature Reviews Microbiology*, vol. 9, March 2011, pp. 244–253, https://doi.org/10.1038/nrmicro2537.

Qiukui Hao, Bi Rong Dong and Taixiang Wu, 'Probiotics for Preventing Acute Respiratory Tract Infections', Cochrane Database of Systematic Reviews, February 2015, https://doi.org/10.1002/14651858.CD006895.pub3.

Yu He et al., 'Main Clinical Features of COVID-19 and Potential Prognostic and Therapeutic Value of the Microbiota in SARS-CoV-2 Infections', *Frontiers in Microbiology*, June 2020, https://doi.org/10.3389/fmicb.2020.01302.

Felice N. Jacka et al., 'A Randomised Controlled Trial of Dietary Improvement for Adults with Major Depression (the "SMILES" trial)', *BMC Medicine*, vol. 15, article 23, January 2017, https://bmcmedicine.biomedcentral.com/articles/10.1186/s12916-017-0791-y.

Wilhelmina Kalt et al., 'Recent Research on the Health Benefits of Blueberries and Their Anthocyanins', *Advances in Nutrition*, vol. 11, no. 2, March 2020, pp. 224–236, https://doi.org/10.1093/advances/nmz065.

Candyce H. Kroenke et al., 'Effects of a Dietary Intervention and Weight Change of Vasomotor Symptoms in the Women's Health Initiative', *Menopause: The Journal of the North American Menopause Society*, vol. 19, no. 9, September 2012, pp. 980–988, https://doi.org/10.1097/gme.0b013e31824f606e.

Derek C. Miketinas et al., 'Fiber Intake Predicts Weight Loss and Dietary Adherence in Adults Consuming Calorie-Restricted Diets: The POUNDS Lost (Preventing Overweight Using Novel Dietary Strategies): A Study', *Journal of Nutrition*, vol. 149, no. 10, October 2019, pp. 1742–1748, https://doi.org/10.1093/jn/nxz117.

Elena Niccolai et al., 'The Gut–Brain Axis in the Neuropsychological Disease Model of Obesity: A Classical Movie Revised by the Emerging Director "Microbiome"', *Nutrients*, vol. 11, no. 1, 2019, p. 156, https://doi.org/10.3390/nu11010156.

K. Rea, T. G. Dinan and J. F. Cryan, 'Gut Microbiota: A Perspective for Psychiatrists', *Neuropsychobiology*, vol. 79, no. 1, February 2020, pp. 50–62, https://doi.org/10.1159/000504495.

Jason M. Ridlon, '*Clostridium scindens*: A Human Gut Microbe with a High Potential to Convert Glucocorticoids into Androgens', *Journal of Lipid Research*, vol. 54, no. 9, September 2013, pp. 2437–2449, https://doi.org/10.1194/jlr.M038869.

Jason Solway et al., 'Diet and Dermatology: The Role of a Whole-Food, Plant-Based Diet in Preventing and Reversing Skin Aging', *Journal of Clinical and Aesthetic Dermatology*, vol. 13, no. 5, May 2020, pp. 38–43, https://www.ncbi.nlm.nih.gov/pmc/articles/PMC7380694/pdf/jcad_13_5_38.pdf.

Hyun Sun-Yoon et al., 'Cocoa Flavanol Supplementation Influences Skin Conditions of Photo-Aged Women: A 24-Week Double-Blind, Randomized, Controlled Trial', *Journal of Nutrition*, vol. 146, no. 1, January 2016, pp. 46–50, https://doi.org/10.3945/jn.115.217711.

Joshua Tarini and Thomas M. S. Wolever, 'The Fermentable Fibre Insulin Increases Postprandial Serum Short-Chain Fatty Acids and Reduces Free-Fatty Acids and Ghrelin in Healthy Subjects', *Applied Physiology, Nutrition, and Metabolism*, January 2020, https://doi.org/10.1139/H09-119.

Christoph A. Thaiss et al., 'Persistent Microbiome Alterations Modulate the Rate of Post-Dieting Weight Regain', *Nature*, vol. 540, 24 November 2016, pp. 544–551, https://www.nature.com/articles/nature20796.

Anne Vrieze et al., 'Transfer of Intestinal Microbiota from Lean Donors Increases Insulin Sensitivity in Individuals with Metabolic Syndrome', *Gastroenterology*, vol. 143, no. 4, October 2012, pp. 913–916.E7, https://doi.org/10.1053/j.gastro.2012.06.031.

Benjamin D. Weger et al., 'The Mouse Microbiome Is Required for Sex-Specific Diurnal Rhythms of Gene Expression and Metabolism', *Cell Metabolism*, vol. 29, no. 2, February 2019, pp. 362–382.E8, https://doi.org/10.1016/j.cmet.2018.09.023.

Inga Wessels and Lothar Rink, 'Micronutrients in Autoimmune Diseases: Possible Therapeutic Benefits of Zinc and Vitamin D', *Journal of Nutritional Biochemistry*, vol. 77, article 108240, March 2020, https://doi.org/10.1016/j.jnutbio.2019.108240.

Marcus White, 'James Lind: The Man Who Helped to Cure Scurvy with Lemons', BBC News, 4 October 2016, https://www.bbc.co.uk/news/uk-england-37320399.

Xuan Zhang et al., 'The Gut Microbiota: Emerging Evidence in Autoimmune Diseases', *Trends in Molecular Medicine*, vol. 26, no. 9, September 2020, pp. 862–873, https://doi.org/10.1016/j.molmed.2020.04.001.

Chapter 5: What's holding you back?

Neal D. Barnard et al., 'A Systematic Review and Meta-Analysis of Changes in Body Weight in Clinical Trials of Vegetarian Diets', *Journal of the Academy of Nutrition and Dietetics*, vol. 115, no. 6, June 2015, pp. 954–969, https://doi.org/10.1016/j.jand.2014.11.016.

Sadie B. Barr and Jonathan C. Wright, 'Postprandial Energy Expenditure in Whole-Food and Processed-Food Meals: Implications for Daily Energy Expenditure', *Food & Nutrition Research*, vol. 54, July 2010, https://doi.org/10.3402/fnr.v54i0.5144.

Julie E. Flood-Obbagy and Barbara J. Rolls, 'The Effect of Fruit in Different Forms on Energy Intake and Satiety at a Meal', *Appetite*, vol. 52, no. 2, April 2009, pp. 416–422, https://doi.org/10.1016/j.appet.2008.12.001.

Kevin D. Hall et al., 'Ultra-Processed Diets Cause Excess Calorie Intake and Weight Gain: An Inpatient Randomized Controlled Trial of *Ad Libitum* Food Intake', *Cell Metabolism*, vol. 30, no. 1, July 2019, pp. 67–77 E3, https://doi.org/10.1016/j.cmet.2019.05.008.

Miguel A. Martínez-González et al., 'A Provegetarian Food Pattern and Reduction in Total Mortality in the PREDIMED Study', *American Journal of Clinical Nutrition*, vol. 100, supplement 1, July 2014, pp. 320S–328S, https://doi.org/10.3945/ajcn.113.071431.

Janet A. Novotny, Sarah K. Gebauer and David J. Baer, 'Discrepancy between the Atwater Factor Predicted and Empirically Measured Energy Values of Almonds in Human Diets', *American Journal of Clinical Nutrition*, vol. 96, no. 2, August 2012, pp. 296–301, https://doi.org/10.3945/ajcn.112.035782.

Hollie A. Raynor et al., 'A Cost-Analysis of Adopting a Healthful Diet in a Family-Based Obesity Treatment Program', *Journal of the Academy of Nutrition and Dietetics*, vol. 102, no. 5, May 2002, pp. 645–656, https://doi.org/10.1016/s0002-8223(02)90148-3.

Chapter 6: The Diversity Diet toolkit

Celia Framson et al., 'Development and Validation of the Mindful Eating Questionnaire', *Journal of the American Diet Association*, author manuscript, August 2010, https://www.ncbi.nlm.nih.gov/pmc/articles/PMC2734460/pdf/nihms136809.pdf.

Donna M. Winham et al., 'Pinto Bean Consumption Reduces Biomarkers for Heart Disease Risk', *Journal of the American College of Nutrition*, vol. 26, no. 3, 2007, pp. 243–249, https://doi.org/10.1080/07315724.2007/10719607.

Recipes

F. De Alzaa et al., 'Evaluation of Chemical and Physical Changes in Different Commercial Oils During Heating', *ACTA Scientific Nutritional Health*, vol. 2, no. 6, June 2018, https://www.actascientific.com/ASNH/pdf/ASNH-02-0083.pdf.

Elli Callegari et al., 'Survival of yogurt bacteria in the human gut', *Appl Environ Microbiol*. 2006 Jul;72(7):5113-7. doi: 10.1128/AEM.02950-05.

Index

Index of Recipes

Acknowledgements

To you guys, The Gut Health Doctor inner community: your heartwarming messages and endless support continue to inspire me every day. Thank you for taking this journey with me.

To Thomas, Claire and Mum, thank you for your brains, energy and support throughout the whole journey; I couldn't have done it without you. To my little Archie, you really were with me every step of the way, from recipe developing and researching (*in utero*) to photo-shooting and editing; thank you for sharing Mummy with this book.

To Sofia, Lucy and Elise, thank you for everything you do for The Gut Health Doctor Community.

To Amy, Hannah, Saffron, Emily, Richard, Alice, Julia, Penguin Life, Andrew, Katie and the shoot team: thank you for sharing your expertise and going that extra mile.

To Jamie and the Jamie Oliver cookery school: thank you for being my pandemic heroes and letting us use your space for recipe testing. You saved my gut microbes and I from a lot of stress!

To my research team at King's College London and all the other researchers whose work I've referenced in this book. Your dedication to science and tireless efforts are truly appreciated.